THE SPIRITUAL
DIMENSIONS
OF *M* USIC

Altering Consciousness for Inner Development

THE SPIRITUAL
DIMENSIONS
OF *M*USIC

Altering Consciousness for Inner Development

R.J. STEWART

Destiny Books
Rochester, Vermont

Destiny Books
One Park Street
Rochester, Vermont 05767
www.DestinyBooks.com

LIBRARY OF CONGRESS CATALOGING-IN-PUBLICATION DATA
Stewart, R.J., 1949–
    [Music and the elemental psyche]
    The spiritual dimensions of music : altering consciousness for
inner development / R.J. Stewart.
        p. cm.
    Originally published under title: Music and the elemental psyche.
    Discography: p.
    Includes bibliographical references and index.
    ISBN 978-0-89281-312-4
    1. Music—Psychology. 2. Music—Philosophy and aesthetics.
I. Title.
ML3830.S84   1990
781'.11–dc20   90–46090
                                                            CIP
                                                            MN

Printed and bound in the United States

10   9   8   7   6

Destiny Books is a division of Inner Traditions International

Contents

Illustrations

Acknowledgements

I would like to express my gratitude to those who directly or indirectly helped with development and expression of the material used in this book: W. G. Gray for introducing me to the system of 'magic squares' in 1969. Basil Wilby for publishing and recording early variants for Helios Bookservice in 1975. Joscelyn Godwin for making the work of Robert Fludd and Fr. Athanasius Kircher available to a wide readership in 1979. Adam Maclean for his interest in the development of the theories in 1982. Felicity Bowers for her superhuman patience in translating my rough sketches into finished artwork in 1985. Appendix 5, part 3, is reproduced by permission of Gareth Knight. I also owe thanks to those who listened to my talks on the subject of metaphysical or alchemical music, and by asking questions helped in the clarification of the theories and the diagrams. But first and last acknowledgement is owed to those Hermetic Philosophers who heard and described the Music of the Spheres, and to the tutelage of Thrice Great Hermes.

Pythagoras reveals the Musical Secret to the Poet

In a quiet place, beneath a spreading Tree,
I sat to rest. Perhaps I fell asleep,
For in a little while appeared to me
A company of Sages rising from the deep
And hidden Earth. Slowly did they pass
Before me with appearance stern,
Led by the Senior of them all, Pythagoras,
Who turned and uttered one word: 'Learn!'

At this command my vision sank Below
Into a Forge where metals were reborn,
And from the anvil every potent blow
Rang with a sound as bright as any horn.
Four Smiths there were who walked the anvil round,
Four brothers of the secret Art;
Each in his turn produced a different sound
Upon a different metal for his part.

Watching them dance, I wondered what was this . . .
Four Smiths, Four Metals, Sixteen Chimes,
A circling and eternal beat;
Until I spied an ancient Sign, the Tetractys,
Inscribed in stone beneath their feet.

Each Number then I counted, adding up to Ten
Wherein Four Only made the Whole,
Whereat the Smiths paused in their work, and when
They paused, a ray of light into that chamber stole.

In through a tiny crack in the dark vault it crept
Growing in strength as if the rising sun
Struck through the earth above. And when it leapt
Reflected from the substance of their Work, it shone,
And as it shone, it Rang and Sounded
Through that Confined Space,
Till daring to look Down, I spied upon the Anvil . . .
My own Face!

At this I woke, and found myself alone,
Sitting upright on the sunlit grass,
While in my hand I clutched a rough old stone
As if it was a looking glass.

R. J. Stewart, 1983

Foreword

This is not a book of comparative musicology; it offers a practical system of musical symbolism which may be applied to change our consciousness. In this sense it is in keeping with the enduring traditions of Western magic and metaphysics, in which music plays a vital part.

No form of communication is as sectarian as music, although it simultaneously acknowledges universality. Before completing this book I circulated copies to various musical experts: one in sound synthesis, one modern serious composer, one academic musicologist, a psychologist and a pop star. Without exception each one became heated over the criticism or presumed criticism offered concerning his or her special field of work. Yet not one of my readers felt that music beyond their own field had been unfairly treated, or at least did not say so. Some of their comments have contributed to the final form of the book, but all content, details and factual matters are my own responsiblity, as are the theories developed throughout the text. I would not wish any of my mistakes to be ascribed to those readers and experts.

Another source of considerable dispute was the Discography; so many conflicting comments were offered by friends and experts regarding the various stages of Discography that I have, with a few exceptions, listed the most up-to-date sources and labels for specialist music, rather than individual titles. There is a trap, into which many modern writers on music and meditation fall, by which descriptions and discographies become mere lists of recordings that cannot by their very nature claim to give the same results in every listener. I have chosen, after much debate, to avoid even approaching this trap. I do not accept that any specific recording can categorically change consciousness . . . but there are traditions of music and changing consciousness which I have attempted to summarize for modern practical use.

(A cassette recording of vocal and instrumental music based on the theories and exercises developed in this book may be obtained from Sulis Music, BCM Box 3721, London WC1N 3XX. This recording includes music on the eighty-stringed concert psaltery, designed by the author in 1970, and featured on a number of albums, stage, film and television productions.)

Introduction

The subject of music and metaphysics is vast, and a short book of this sort is essentially and deliberately limited. My main reason for writing was the surprising lack of any direct method in publication that offered musical alchemy, therapy or elemental psychic mapping to the general reader.

When I first became aware of metaphysical and psychological traditions within music, traditions that were known at least as far back as the sixth century BC in Greece, it soon became clear that there were a large number of books on the subject. These ranged from academic studies and sources, to long complex treatises and Renaissance theosophical expositions. Modern studies had been produced by philosophers and esoteric researchers such as Rudolph Steiner, and many of the major books on magic and metaphysics included sections on music. The major sources were often untranslated from their Latin originals, and even in translation were difficult to apply; they could be studied, compared, and summarized in the usual scholarly manner, but there seemed to be very little that the budding metaphysical musician could actually *do*. This was in spite of the infuriating knowledge that practical applications lay just below the surface, ready to leap forth if only the right key could be found to liberate them from their recondite intellectual bondage.

At the opposite extreme to the source works and great philosophers or metaphysicians were a number of derivative popular books. These seemed to copy uncritically and often inaccurately from the larger reference sources, inevitably without any deeper understanding of the principles that lay behind the systems of correspondence. In so-called esoteric music, as in most popular books on 'occultism' authors happily and naïvely copied one another, generating the most absurd nonsense and vesting it with a spurious hierarchical gravity. Most of the lightweight studies of esoteric music followed a historical or supposedly evolutionary pattern, leaving the reader to wonder what, if anything, generated this pattern or enlivened it. We were never given any hint on proper use or development of metaphysical music within ourselves . . . as if it was not the property of mankind in general but a subject best left to the angels, hierarchies or withdrawn secret masters who were supposed to direct human evolution and inspire certain utterly average composers.

I boldly embarked upon a book called *Music and Magic* as early as 1971; but it soon became clear that this would read like any of the other lightweight books on the subject, and since those early days a number of derivative and all too familiar books on music and metaphysics have appeared, copying from other writers.

It is, in fact, very difficult to write a book on music and consciousness without retracing ground already covered but never vitalized sufficiently to fire the reader's imagination. This is not because there is too little to say, but because it is surprisingly difficult to express the material intellectually in print. My hasty sense of frustration with the published sources, both great and small, gradually became one of sympathy for the authors . . . excluding, perhaps, the mere copyists and mystery-mongers. The task of communicating metaphysical or magical or psychological music to the reader is not an easy one, especially as much of the root material has traversed many centuries of cultural change and is expressed in language and concepts now almost alien to the modern mind.

I resolved to return to basics, to attempt that which had been attempted by earlier writers of Hermetic theories, and express the material in the language of my own day, with a series of simple illustrations. But it was not until a workable musical map or open-ended system appeared that I seriously considered scrapping my original manuscript and starting afresh. The results are the theory and psycho-musical experiment found in the following chapters and their diagrams.

A very limited edition of my *Elemental Music* theory was published by the now defunct Helios Bookservice in Great Britain in 1974-5. This was in the form of notes for a set of magical/musical recordings now out of print and probably superseded by later material from the various writers involved. During the ten-year period between the appearance of those original notes and the writing of this book, I worked repeatedly with the system described, and found that it could be demonstrated easily and clearly at public lectures. There are a number of developments and applications which are not included here, which apply mainly to instrumental music and the relationship between vocal, instrumental music and sacred dance. I hope that these subjects will form the basis for a future book.

1.

Music and Changing Consciousness

The contents of this book are drawn from my own experience as a composer and musician, and as a researcher into the more unusual aspects of music. It is essentially a short practical book . . . a handbook of musical alchemy, if we use an old-fashioned but still viable description. There is no suggestion, however, of quaintness obscurity or wilful confusion, such as is sometimes found in books that deal mysteriously with the Hermetic sciences. I am concerned with a set of simple concepts, application of specific theories, and a modern method of alternative involvement with music of all sorts. Alternative is used here in its proper sense, and not as a banner for fashionable escapism.

This is not an academic book, and it may be used by the general reader and enthusiast as easily as by the composer or musician, the acoustician or scholar of early musical development. The practical alternatives of musical involvement may also be applied on a different level, by the modern meditator or group seeking to make willed changes in consciousness through use of specific musical theories and selected examples of music. This application ranges from musical therapy to spiritual disciplines.

The theories outlined, therefore, should hold something for everyone interested in the possibilities of Music and Changing Consciousness . . . they are not confined to any one specialist area, but are intended to bridge a number of disciplines and musically operative systems or concepts. Most important of all I hope to demonstrate that some extremely simple conceptual models, which were central to earlier cultures, can still have a modern and dynamic application today, transformed within the context of our rapidly changing and fragmented societies worldwide. As the material is written specifically for the Western reader, however, it does not include any oriental musical terminology, nor does it demand that we make the quite false assumption that the West has no truly magical music of its own. This subject is dealt with in detail elsewhere in the book, and need not be taken any further here.

To gain the best results from this book you do not have to be a musician, a psychologist or even a magician . . . but you do have to be seriously interested in music as a genuine power that effects changes in consciousness. These changes can be the ephemeral moods of the individual as he or she drifts willy-nilly across the commercial musical landscape, or they may be profound long-term effects that interlink with vast cycles of social and economic transformation.

More rarely, but most significant of all, music may also generate dynamic and permanent changes in the individual consciousness, be it saint, poet, composer, or a less specifically defined seeker after reality and truth, a musical everyman or woman. These changes arise from combinations of frequencies and patterns that resonate equally for the physicist as for the metaphysicist, albeit in different worlds.

The resonances are utilized by an ancient, enduring, but easily confused set of artistic sciences, of which alchemy, magic, and theosophy or metaphysics form a major part. In such artistic sciences, of which modern psychology is a direct descendant despite its limitations, the inner perceptions, intuitions and revelations of highly sensitized persons are combined with painstaking practical work and well-established conceptual models. I say easily confused not because the artistic sciences are inherently difficult or jumbled, but because as moderns we approach them from the outside and try to break through into their heart. Like any true discipline they may only be operated from within, after arduous training, and nobody likes the thought of such hard labour today.

As with all such systems or disciplines, however, there are a small number of 'direct approaches' which can speed up the more obvious results. They are like crash-diets, health and fitness training or purgatives, and are found in the catalytic methods of magic and psychotherapy.[1] Music cuts across this problem, and forms a link between the long tedious discipline and the cathartic inner transformation induced suddenly. In other words, music makes life better through its own inherent power — with the important proviso that we must control the music, and not let the music of would-be controllers control us!

The combination of intuitive vision and practical discipline runs through primal, magical, liturgical, meditational and alchemical music, and reappears today in the various systems of music therapy proliferating out of materialist pyschology. As this modern movement of music and psychotherapy, or music and its holistic effect upon human vitality, is directly related to the old magical and alchemical musical systems (though it usually is ignorant of them or wilfully chooses not to acknowledge their existence), I have included a short but eclectic list of reference works. This list forms the basis for the notes to each chapter, within a longer Bibliography for further reading.

The acoustics expert or the musicologist with a firm understanding of the physics of music, particularly in the context of early music and historical changes, may find correlations in the systems which are offered here, correlations that are not included in my own explanations or suggestions for the general reader, as they are matters of fine technical distinction which do not affect the practical application of music to consciousness. This technical matter raises the important question of material dissection versus a conceptual overview. I doubt if we can really find the secret heart of music by examination of its physics, its acoustic history or its theoretical mathematics, which are so different from its actual use by human beings.

Many other short books on music, magic and changing consciousness precede this one, plus a number of large and profound volumes by monumental thinkers, metaphysicians, physicists and theologians or theosophists. The subject has an enduring fascination, for it attunes to the depths of human awareness and our intuitions about reality, truth and communication. Most of the shorter and more recent books have tried to correlate the history of music (usually in Europe but occasionally drawing upon oriental cross-references) through the concept of evolution. They take a historical-cultural framework, and cite individual composers as examples of an evolving musical consciousness, which reaches into the present day (of the author of each book). I do not subscribe to this view of music, and do not attempt to formulate the development of music in this manner.[2]

To define human consciousness in music through specific composers, theorists or musical works is quite inadequate; it confines our understanding to a false temporal progression in which the illusion of social evolution or material evolution and scientific progress is confused with an equally false notion of musical evolution.

While art music appears, superficially, to evolve through definable stages, such stages are only truly apparent in retrospect. Though it seems innocently logical on the surface, retrospective analysis which is guided by the concept of evolution always generates a false picture of progress. This fallacy is more obvious when we look at retrospective analyses of prophecies and predictions, where obscure utterances are crammed intellectually into historical contexts which are only valid by hindsight rather than by inspiration.[3] The evolutionary picture is so firmly interwoven with the concepts of scientific and social progress that other modes of *progression*, which may be spiral or oblique, are ignored.[4] This is particularly noticeable in our histories of music, be they mainstream or fringe studies, where certain key persons, theories, works, or technical developments are highlighted in an unnatural manner. While such powerful innovations undoubtedly occur, they do so upon a vast protean background of musical activity and common consciousness, most of which is quite unaffected by the fashions of art music, and lives according to patterns or rules which I outline in brief as part of the main argument of this book. I should stress that we are not talking about 'folk-music' in this context, but about human-consciousness-music, of which folk or ethnic music plays only one important part in a spiralling musical work of timeless duration.

Many writers on the subject of music suggest that we are about to move into an age of great freedom, in which the undeniably strangling restrictions of European art music are being broken down, in which musical freedom is gained through the use of highly sophisticated instruments which will generate pleromas of sound.[5] Yet such pleromas or whole-sounds have always been with us, in our voices, or in the simplest of musical instruments, if we choose to hear them. Technology is not necessarily a sign of musical progress, though it can make a superb servant.

Far from suggesting that we are about to swing into a musical new age, I suspect that future generations, applying retrospective analysis to prove how advanced their own music is by comparison to ours, will see the twentieth and twenty-first centuries as the nadir in the devolution of music within human consciousness. I think that music holds a potency now almost but not quite lost to us, and that there are certain plummeting low points in our musical 'development' which must be rebalanced socially and individually for psychic and physical well-being. I do not suggest that we should try to escape into a spurious musical past, but that we must find a way of dealing with the paradoxical relationship between musical devolution and spiralling changes of consciousness.

The general directions of my theories is not pessimistic, but regenerative. We should, above all, find a way of stepping back from some extremely debilitating stereotypes found within both art and popular music, to enable us to judge what, if anything, is really happening to modern musical development. It is in this context, initially, that the old Hermetic or ancient metaphysical systems are useful as psychological correctives. They must not be taken at face value, as they are expressed through orthodox religious or philosophical symbolism which is repellent to many modern minds; but we may seek out the perennial core of their systems, and state it in simple and unambiguous ways. One such way or model forms a main part of this book, and I strongly encourage the reader to try it out, for it has not yet been known to fail if genuine unbiased effort is put into honest experimentation.

There is little doubt in my mind, but also little proof in the academic historical sense, that the alchemists and Hermetic philosophers drew upon musical traditions that extend back into the cultures of the distant past. The obvious influences of Greece, Rome and the Arabic cultures are well known and demonstrated in popular studies of alchemy,[6] and in recent years increasing proof of native Western European lore and symbolism has been brought forward by various scholars and authors.[7] The system of musical metaphysics which I demonstrate in the later chapters is as likely to have been used by the Celtic Druids as it was by the Pythagorean Greeks, but the musical evidence for this suggestion is rooted in the folk music and remnants of bardic lore from Ireland, Wales, Scotland and Brittany.[8]

Ultimately, magical, alchemical or metaphysical music, which is music that has a psycho-logical application, must have a grounding in the essential nature of the psyche, of consciousness itself. It is facile to suggest that all music is grounded in this way; by doing so I would be withdrawing behind a true statement that is so diffused and general that no one individual could really attempt to apply it. We are all familiar with such grandiose but ineffective 'wisdom' teachings, and really need to get our teeth into something hard, particular and, of course, nutritious. Any good musical and psycho-musical system must lead us out of generality into a specific, then back to the generality which is now seen to be transformed. If the route taken is complex, obscure, obtuse and perhaps elitist, we should not take it.

I hope that the theories, methods, clues and maps offered here are a start, a move towards a clarity in applied music-consciousness which will be taken and improved by later and better people. As I have followed and simplified an enduring core tradition, so I am certain that others will continue with the same alchemical process of refinement and transformation.

Systems and Diagrams
Before embarking upon the routes shown by the musical and metaphysical maps in the text and diagrams, I would ask the reader not to become too entrapped within 'Systems'. There is no intention on my

part of offering a system or systems supposedly 'authoritative' or 'definitive'. The best that can be said for any system is that it is (a) effective in doing what it claims to do, and (b) that it leads to its own demolition via the liberation of those who employ it to reach new conclusions, fresh insights, and real inner or outer growth.

The fallacy of authoritative systems, or even worse, occult and elitist systems, is our unfortunate conceptual inheritance from an orthodox dogmatic male-dominated religion. It runs through all levels of European-American culture, but in this context we are concerned with its corruption of the power of music and magic in human consciousness.

Many esoteric works are elitist and dogmatic, even those claiming to carry us beyond the formal Church or apparently in opposition to decaying religion. Most of these books are written by men and occasionally women — who were heavily conditioned by the orthodox Church . . . and in the case of writers prior to the twentieth century were often members of the priesthood. Within this false ambience of 'authority', maintained by force of arms where necessary, is the image of the patriarch, an all-wise domineering male who utters 'truths' that are 'definitive'.

In more recent times, this image has appeared as the epitome of 'reason'; authority is defined by a mania for proof or experimental validity. In magic, music, and in the human psyche, proof is frequently transcended, and reason continually sidestepped in favour of deeper levels of understanding which are not accessible to verbal or intellectual definition. In psychology we still find this image of rampant or demonic stereotypical male wisdom, where all facets of the human entity are falsely defined through various schools of reductionism or superficial labelling.

In music it is the composer, of course, who carries this stereotype, often unwittingly or unwillingly. The illusion of one person, usually male, through whom creative impulses are frozen upon paper in unyielding and unchangeable form (the score) is one that becomes less and less valid for musical maturity in society, but nevertheless retains enormous power. In popular music the power is expressed as income, stardom, and an almost religious intensity of devotion from fans, but this degraded area of mass conditioning is, curiously, one of the crossing points that leads us back to a more imaginative approach to music. It is a corrupted path, however, as it adds to the devolution of our shared imagination, triggered by trivialities and crude ploys to generate sales.

To balance this unfortunate male stereotype, we must remember that the magical, esoteric and subsequent alchemical or Hermetic writings and teachings retained a vast inheritance from the pagan cults and ancient philosophies. These were intimately involved with the image and regenerative powers of a goddess or goddesses, the female elements rejected or corrupted by Christianity. The Roman Church, however, restored this female image in the form of the cult of the Virgin, thus attempting to absorb the energies of the pagan goddess images which were still at large in the common imagination.[9]

The curious systems, mainly shown here in simple diagram form, are partly derived from pre-Christian philosophy and metaphysics. Such conceptual models appeared in various cultures, including classical Greece and the influential Eastern sources who contributed so much to the growth of Christianity. We receive this material through the filtering of the rampant censorship and distortion of the political Churches, but also retain it in various traditional forms handed down at very general cultural levels — through folklore, poetry, song, ritual dance and other elements which slid under, so to speak, the barriers set up by orthodoxy. The alchemical writings from the middle ages through to the eighteenth century show a strong influence of such traditions upon individual thinkers and mystics, while a number of important medieval texts from native traditions, perhaps originally Druidic Celtic, also offer us evidence of symbolic continuity.[10]

The systems are *open-ended*; they are fluid, accomodating, flexible. They are not rigid or authoritarian; you will not fail in any way if you do not follow them precisely. Indeed, magical, psychological and metaphysical topologies change immediately when they are energized by human consciousness. In music, a composer's rigid marks upon paper come alive by the recreation of the musical vision at the interpretation of a conductor and in the hands of a great musician or group of musicians. This is an obvious example of a psychic topology (the score) coming alive and changing through human consciousness.

The formal maps in our diagrams, such as the *Tree of Life* or the *Fourfold Elemental System* appear to be constant or even rigid to the superficial examination, but once they are enlivened by deeper imaginative attention, vital changes occur within their living matrices.

The concepts suggested, therefore, are not a set of systems that will replace or revolutionize anything that already claims to be definitive or fixed; they are a family of matrices, mother-images which will help our impoverished musical awareness towards belated adulthood. We cannot use these systems to 'compose' in the usual sense of the word, though I have created and recorded music by applying some of the principles described.[11] The non-systems illustrated should help us to rid ourselves of the false limitations of musical authority at one extreme (art music) and to guard ourselves against chaotic fragmentation at the other (popular music).

What happens after that is very much up to the individual, to yourself.

The diagrams are made as simple and direct as possible and may be used in several different ways. They are not intended to improve upon the remarkable and imaginative maps of correspondences found in earlier works (such as those of the great metaphysicians like Fludd or Kircher),[12] but to demonstrate the barest essentials of such maps devoid of complex attributes. There are a number of original diagrams, based upon the ancient model of the Four Elements, which have not been published before, as they are the results of my own musical/alchemical system described in the main text. The functions of the diagrams are as follows:

1. To clarify concepts discussed in the text.
2. To provide simple keys to the more complex diagrams found in earlier books on metaphysics, magic and music.[13]
3. To state a number of theories and concepts in the old traditional manner (such as the Lyre of Apollo, the Instrument with Four Strings, or the Musical Man).
4. To act as visual symbols for contemplation, meditation, or concentration aided by imagination. In this role the diagrams move out of the merely intellectual dimensions into those of the inner disciplines or magical or mystical arts.
5. To act as psychic topologies, linked not only to (4) above, but to the general matrix used for mapping the human psyche in the ancient philosophies. This matrix, the Fourfold Pattern, generates many other more complex topological glyphs, such as the Tree of Life, the Platonic Solids, and in physics the maps by which early realizations of the structure of the solar system were made concrete. It is worth stressing that such maps are not outmoded curiosities, but can still be used very effectively by the modern student of the psyche.[14]
6. To demonstrate the perennial concept that there is a harmonic relationship between the *microcosm* — humankind, and the *macrocosm* — the universe. Strictly speaking we may apply this term macrocosm to the solar system only, as the greater universe is yet another harmonic level, which could be called the hypercosm.
7. To demonstrate, in the case of the elemental glyph diagrams (Chapter 5), a direct relationship between modes of consciousness and musical shapes. By this simple method, we remove music from the linear progression of the time-bound notation system, and demonstrate it upon the elemental map of consciousness used in ancient psychology and metaphysics. As all such circular maps are

flat analogies of a spherical geometry, we are also creating an analogical model to link musical vibrations with more abstract mathematics.

This mathematical direction is not developed in our text, as it obviously belongs in a more technical work, but the analogy may be taken through the usual stages: 'flat' 'spherical' and multi-dimensional. It is possible to use this system to define music in any number of mathematical dimensions, and musical creation can be dramatically enlivened by application of this type of analogy.

The models shown are only the most basic, and a large series of other maps or conceptual glyphs could be added to this first collection. I would like to stress that however fascinating the mathematical combinations or rotations are, they cannot replace the inner application or meditation upon the original Fourfold Pattern from which they all derive.

If we were to spend our time researching the mathematics, rotations, combinations and formulae generated by the theories described, we would be missing the point. In the musical models of Renaissance philosophers, the mathematical truths were used to demonstrate metaphysical truths, following the Hermetic axiom of 'as above so below'. The physics or mathematics were never intended as ends in themselves, merely as suggestive modes of mental activity which attuned to higher consciousness.

My approach in this book is similar, but very basic. No attempt is made to use physics or mathematics to 'prove' anything; the geometric analogies shown in the diagrams are closely derived from a set of primary creative concepts, shown in metaphysics and astrology as the Four Elements or the Four Worlds. These, as I state in a later chapter, are *states of relative activity* which may be used to define both inner and outer phenomena, applicable to both physics and metaphysics, the society and the psyche. Beyond these, mystics relate the existence of another state, which cannot be defined in relative terms, and is accessible only through meditation. Our musical analogies do not touch upon this state, but assuredly derive from it, even if we as individuals may never realize it fully.[14]

If we discard all historical, intellectual and mathematical derivatives we are left with a set of symbols, such as those shown in our diagrams. These may be considered directly, in their own right, and they have certain inherent qualities which resonate within the human psyche and biological organism. If you approach them in a very direct and uncomplicated manner, you will bring them alive, and also bring alive those harmonic powers of your own psyche and body which are intimately attuned to music.[15]

For many of us, simple exercises of the sort described will be our first experience with conscious use of music upon our minds and bodies. Most musical experience is passive, often to an extent of passivity that would never be acceptable in any other type of life activity. Our consumption of music is directly comparable to that of a person lying flat upon his or her back, and allowing unknown others to pour unknown substances into the stomach through a funnel. We then wonder why our sense of *taste* is so confused, why we are *undernourished*, and why we are often drugged, poisoned and generally weakened.

By regarding music as a power for changing consciousness, we first close our mouths to random or compulsive intake. This in itself is no small task, but is aided by the hard fact that we must make a choice: do we allow others to pump us full of product or artful contrivance, or do we, perhaps for the first time in our lives, try to contact some of the inner fundamentals behind the power of music?

At a later stage we select our own musical nourishment very carefully, following and improving upon the dietary hints in Appendix 1. In time, and with effort, we can change ourselves from mere consumers drugged upon pap, or artistic stereotypes supported by fashion, and eventually stand upon our own feet as musically alert individuals.

Obviously my analogy is deliberately overstated, but if it makes you in any way uncomfortable with your own musical intake, it is likely to have some truth for you. I would stress that this analogy applies to the composer and musician as well as to the non-musician, though in the case of the specialist the diet is more likely to be one of excess of one or two specific musical elements, and absence of sympathy in experience of others.

In a culture where music is pumped from every room, shop, cafe and public gathering place, the proposition of controlled intake may seem wildly idealistic. How do we stop the flood of garbage that assails us from every loudspeaker? It is clear, but perhaps regrettable, that we are not allowed to take instant direct action against music pollution. Axes are socially inadmissible and dangerous to innocent bystanders, while electronic interference with broadcasting signals is illegal in most countries.

The elemental exercises offered here have a number of effects, one of which is the gradual ability to de-tune (not ignore or merely shut out) the effect of unwanted music. In the case of strong and debilitating rhythms, such as that used in rock music, some of our exercises may even be used in the traditional manner of the focus, prayer or mantram, where they literally cut across unwanted influences. This is, however, rather a drastic application of musical symbols which are really intended for more profound prolonged development.

In this context we must remember that the value is one of musical consciousness, of music that we employ within our psyche, and not one of external expression. I am not suggesting that we all go around chanting the vocal exercises of the Elements at the tops of our voices (though this might be fun), but that we use the *patterns* as emergency correctives in musically distasteful situations. Even visualizing the glyphs or symbols (Chapters 5 and 6) has a surprisingly beneficial effect upon the consciousness weakened by the noise of disco music or the spiritually depressing sounds of certain modern composers.

Ultimately, the musically healthy psyche is able to merely detach itself from such unhealthy influences, but this is a very difficult ideal that involves considerable work upon the unity of the body and the psyche. I would stress the work upon the physical organism, as music is a *physical* power, not emotional, intellectual or spiritual alone. The body reacts directly to certain resonances, pitches and rhythms, a simple fact well known and demonstrated in orthodox science and medicine. These reactions are so complex, however, that it is difficult to control or define them in a rational or ordered manner.

The metaphysical or psychic musical systems offer an alternative method of operation, in which the direct physical response to music is monitored and guided by an inner analogy rather than by outwardly 'proven' rules or experiments. By using such a method, we also bypass certain gross or destructive aspects of music research, such as the dangerous frequencies used to induce physical reactions as a result of brain activity stimulated by sonic triggers.

In the ancient philosophies the physical and spiritual are not separate but are intimately interlinked. Music, a physical pattern of energy apparent in the outer world, demonstrates certain spiritual patterns of energy normally accessible only through highly developed inner perceptions. We can bypass all of this theory, and merely apply its models to our own musical consciousness. As our musical consciousness is harmonically attuned to our entire entity, healthy use of music will stimulate a healthy body.

The statement of health is no mere generalization, for conductors who are exposed to and intimately involved with a wide spectrum of music tend to be healthy and active in advanced old age. This is due as much to the physical contact with musical frequencies upon the entire organism (blasted by a wide range of tones for many years) as it is to the theoretical and artistic or emotional content of the conductor's work.[16] I would suggest that the elemental theory of music expressed in the following pages gives a possible explanation for this musically and biologically proven vitality. There is, of course, the proviso that we must lead a generally healthy and non-self-abusive life. No amount of the best music in the world will fully activate a bloodstream full of drugs, alcohol or the accumulated toxins of an unhealthy diet. Musical stimuli, however, may help us to kick certain bad habits, and the Elemental musical signals can be employed directly for mild therapy in this manner.

Future Developments

I have freely rambled through a number of topics either directly pertinent to the main text and its use by the reader, or to the general subject of music and changing consciousness. To carry any one of these various topics further demands a specialist book of its own, and also demands discipline and individual work beyond the scope of this general exposition. Many of the areas touched upon are extremely fruitful for further development, and it is worth outlining these once more, before we proceed to the theory itself.

1. *Therapy.* Music has been known to be therapeutic from the most distant times, and in early cultures it was not a mere entertainment as it is today. The therapeutic value of specific application of music extends far beyond mere inducement of 'moods', for there are physical reactions within the body when it contacts the physical emissions of controlled sound, i.e. music. The Elemental system outlined will repay simple therapeutic work, and may be operated in several different ways:
   (a) As recorded sonics for passive reception.
   (b) As vocal chants for active inner musical changing of consciousness. This method will affect the organism both inwardly and outwardly, building up a mutual resonance (technically called feedback) which has considerably more power than the original sound signal itself.
   (c) As meditational or magical/spiritual exercises for the dedicated mystic or metaphysician. This is the most specialized application.
   (d) As visual material. The glyphs or charts have a therapeutic or changing influence upon consciousness, even without the sonic symbols being uttered. This is no more than a restatement of the ancient art of the glyph, visual symbol or mandala, known to have psychically therapeutic value. [17]

2. *Communication.* Music is our highest form of communication, though it is frequently degraded to an extremely impoverished level. There

are implications within the concept of *Spherical Music* that could change composition, performance and communication through live music. The emphasis here is on *live* music, though recorded material is an acceptable second best in musical metaphysics. Communication is usually divided into the roles of:

(a) active and outgoing;

(b) passive and receptive.

These roles are defined in music by the performer and the listener, but such an analysis only holds up to superficial reason, and does not work upon the inner or psychic levels of the human entity. There are a number of complex interactions in music, which are shown in potential by the Tree of Life, a polarity diagram of considerable sophistication.

The archetypical musical patterns (Elemental calls or chants) may be employed for levels of communication that transcend verbal intellectual message systems. This is not a wild claim, for we do this regularly in general music, where a composer encapsulates a message, an emotion, an intuition, into his or her musical work, and sends it through time and space to the listener, via the medium of the psyche and body of the performer. Put simply, certain tunes and songs are sad, happy, depressing, vitalizing, and so forth.

In religious monastic use worldwide, chants are seeded with powerful inner or spiritual communication. This may be in the form of dogmatic texts, primal vowel sounds, or specially assembled structures based upon metaphysical 'alphabets'. Many of these topics are discussed in the following pages, and they are all areas of communication which could be developed by modern workers, removing them from the dogmatic or spuriously hierarchical atmosphere that surrounds them.

Communication is Therapy

The therapeutic value of music and the communicative value are merely different manifestations of one mediating and transformative energy. When we practise the traditional types of chant exercise we are, initially, communicating to different areas of levels of our own *entity*. This stage is therapeutic, for it reawakens our 'dead' physical and psychic interactions through the musical stimulus.

On more advanced levels, a truly transformative or spiritual impulse may be communicated from one being to another. Hence the brief but glorious insights provided by some types of religious or mystical music, for such music temporarily (within time-limits) raises our imagination and our physical response to modes of energy and consciousness that we cannot normally sustain.

In magical arts, this communication is extended to link up various realms, worlds and beings which are traditionally said to exist. This type of activity seems less important and valuable, however, than a clear and simple spiritual insight from within. The exercises in this book are not intended for use in superficial or curious conjuration.[18]

Such a role, that of a bridge between worlds, may play an important part in the music of the future; our science reveals more and more of the depths of material existence, and the musical models of the ancient cultures may one day provide the basis for new areas of experiment, models of the universe, or communication with states of being, or self-aware beings, which we cannot at present comprehend. This is not an ignorant reversion to superstition, but a mere suggestion that musical models can act as carriers of signals into dimensions which may not be accessible through any other practical means. As the patterns of musical emission are said, traditionally, to carry the imprint of the original Word, or creative impulse, or origin of all being, they are used metaphysically to act as a universal language that transcends all spaces, times and events. The human response to music is merely one minute Microcosmic aspect of a response and utterance that runs harmonically through the Macrocosm (a star or solar system) and the Hypercosm (the entirety of existence, the universe).

Having extrapolated or intuitively reached thus far, we begin to enter the realms of poetry and of prophecy, of vision that coalesces within regular consciousness, of inspiration that might be expressed as music. The colourful medieval *Prophecies of Merlin*, probably drawn from an ancient Celtic set of verses, describe the end of the solar system at their conclusion: 'The Four Winds shall fight together with a dreadful blast and the sound shall reach the stars'. This is an apocalyptic or dramatic way of describing the interaction of the Four Elements, shown in our main text to be the basis for all musical expression. We find a similar vision in the Creation of the Worlds described in the *Vita Merlini*, a mystical biography drawing upon mixed classical and Druidic or British motifs, also from the pen of twelfth-century chronicler (or assembler) Geoffrey of Monmouth: 'Out of nothing the Creator of the world produced four elements that they might be the prior cause as well as the material for creating all things when they are joined together in harmony . . .'[19] A similar vision is found in Plato's *Republic*, which is quoted in Appendix 2.

I do not cite these ancient writings, to which a large number of other examples may be freely added, as 'sources' or 'authorities'; they are examples of a perpetual mode of perception which exists within ourselves.[20] This mode or pattern of consciousness tends towards archetypes, which are (contrary to the modern rather weak misuse of the term) matrices through which innumerable but harmonically related images, energies and events may be expressed into time and space. When we set these archetypes out in words or in diagramatic form, one of their main presentations is as glyphs, simple charts or geometric maps. Other presentations are also possible, in more anthropomorphic or visionary form, but such expressions are usually a second or derivative stage of symbolism as it ferments its way outwards through the psyche towards material expression.

It is significant that the classical and Renaissance visions or archetypical plans all involve not only music in this world but the spiritual power of music as a universal creative power. We do not experience music in this way today, and so are surprised by correlations between music and therapy, insight and transcendent vision or communication. To work towards a rejuvenation of our musical perceptions, to come alive in those potent imaginative realms beyond gross materialism, we must return to some very simple primary foundations.

2.

Four Ages of Music

Music is a potent power which can alter our awareness. This relationship between music and consciousness, both in the individual and the group, has been known from ancient times. Today it is effectively applied in the widespread commercial exploitation of recorded and broadcast entertainment. Yet despite this acknowledged power of music, it would be unusual for a modern composer or player to clearly describe the root causes of the effective changes that arise within the listener.

Superficially this lack of theoretical approach to music and changing consciousness is part of the growth of simplistic materialism; music is no longer defined in religious terms, so there is less need to relate it to outmoded concepts of divinity. Frequently music is discussed in emotional or so-called 'subjective' terms, or in a rational structural manner which often avoids the primal musical function — that of living communication.

In most historic periods of musical fashion and developments, music is generated by an interaction between listening groups (the public or patrons) and individual creators. This interaction rapidly crystallizes as sets of formulae. We can detect this process immediately in popular music, where the formulae are crude and repetitive, and so dehumanized that recordings are freely referred to as 'product'. Music has become a factory output, part of the great flood of product that includes both tranquillizers and television sets, soap powder and instant soup.

Such mechanistic production of music reflects an overall condition of our culture, manifesting through electronic synthesis, recording and playback equipment. But we should not glamorize the product of past eras merely because it was not amplified or massively broadcast.

The so-called classical music of the eighteenth and nineteenth centuries in Europe reflected the rigid formal culture of the patronizing classes.

It was as replete with production formulae as any twentieth-century ditty programmed through a digital computer keyboard. We might extend this rather unkind analysis of music as product backwards in time until we lose both sight and sound, and arrive at the mysterious music created by our ancestors in the prehistoric past.

No dissection of form, style or presentation in performance or recording can touch upon the secret heart of music, the heart that emits a power which can alter our awareness. This power of change can seem emotional, intellectual, spiritual or sexual, simply because music acts as a vehicle for modes of awareness that both transcend and underpin our normal patterns of consciousness. Music can reinforce these patterns, or, more rarely, it can break them down. This effect is clearly seen again in popular music, where the product moulds and reinforces the ephemeral commercially stereotyped values of the consumer, yet may be intensely irritating and disturbing to members of a different group. While music acts in this manner in the broad fields of commercialism, such effects indicate the extreme potency that may be inherent in highly energized and refined musical vehicles, and it is this rare type of music that we shall explore and begin to experience.

Traditionally such music was transferred by individual tuition, sometimes between humans and Otherworld tutors, as in the fairy music taught in Celtic countries. We shall return to some of these ancient concepts in our later chapters, for they are not mere superstition but are a simple expression of musical power inherent in nature — both human and non-human.

Through the customary intellectual analysis of music we may glean fascinating insights into the personal creativity of great composers; we can often recognize in retrospect that specific works reflect key periods of national or cultural entity and development. In both of these contexts music has a magical or invocatory role closely allied to the arousal and shaping of group emotion, seeded by one visionary source — the composer. Such an attitude to music is typically European, and is of quite recent origin and currency. It may reach profound depths of primal imagery and energy, as in Stravinsky's 'Rite of Spring'; it may climb to aery mathematical rotations of order, as in the works of Bach; or it may remain upon the meanest product level, wherein the sole aim is to sell plastic discs of forgettable songs.

We could add other categories and examples to our list, which is not meant to be definitive in any way. Of particular interest in the context of music and changing consciousness is the fact that our third sample category (commercial popular music) is superficially trivial, but inwardly potent. It can be a most effective tool for shaping individual and group response. Furthermore, unless a countering or negative response is truly active within the listener, popular music will lull and titillate the would be 'classicist' or 'modernist' as easily as it works upon the young consumer at whom it is aimed. Those with affirmed interest in 'better' forms of music may deny this effect, but only until they find themselves tapping their feet to a loud radio playing in the street or humming a crude melodic phrase overheard from a television commercial.

Paradoxically it is at this gross and trivial level that we find the magical power of music, as opposed to the much lauded individual creativity of the serious composer which is not expressed to society at large. The remarkable and invaluable phenomenon of formal individual composition has tended to disguise the true power of music as an impersonal *physical* power that intimately re-attunes human consciousness. This impersonal power is a property of nature, is recognized in the ancient music of the East, and is still potent in many streams of musical expression in the West. Although we have used popular music as the most glaring example on the crudest level, it is by no means the only example, and we shall encounter an enduring tradition of magical music which alters awareness, a tradition which is primarily Western in its origin and preservation.

Due to lamentable ignorance and wilful miseducation, Westerners think that they have no inherent magical music in their culture, and that all 'magic' comes from the individual composer, often in the working out of his or her emotional crises. As we shall discover, there is an enduring and effective set of Western traditions for music that changes consciousness; this teaching has survived from the most distant past right into the present day, and it still works.[1]

The Four Ages of Music and Consciousness

To approach the magical/musical traditions, we must first define a basic progression of musical development. The musical and metaphysical systems of the West are based upon a Fourfold matrix, within which computations of five, seven, ten and twelvefold patterns are developed. We shall return to this simple but far-reaching concept repeatedly during our discussion and examination of metaphysical or transformative music. We shall also encounter a set of exercises for personal or group use, in which musical phrases or calls are used for changing consciousness. Before attempting these exercises, however, the basic fourfold matrix should be understood, and it expresses itself in a number of different ways with regard to music, individual and collective consciousness, and cultural development.[2]

Initially we can identify 'Four Ages' of Music and Consciousness.

1. Primal

Primal music appears from the inspired use of sound sources in nature. *Individually* this manifests as the human voice; *culturally* as primitive music-making activities and inventions. These include singing or chanting, shouting, and a large range of simple but surprisingly versatile instruments. Examples of such instruments are known from archaeological and anthropological evidence, and include whistles, scrapers, drums and many others sources of sound generation. Some of the instruments are ascribed speculatively, or by comparison to modern primitive examples, but they all derive from natural sources. Modern primitives are known to create vocal tones of great beauty and skill, and to create instruments from natural sources such as reeds, branches, stones or skins quite spontaneously. In some cases the instrument is disposed of after it has been played, while in others it acquires a magical significance and identity and is preserved honourably.

2. Environmental

Environmental or ethnic folk music represents a development of the primal use of musical sound. It has a culturally unique quality intimately related to the land of origin. It is this quality which makes folk music instantly recognizable; the music of Spain or of Scotland for example, lives, each having a separate entity of shape, spirit and imaginative tradition. Such musics can never be confused with one another, although detailed study of folk music from a variety of countries reveals many close parallels. In the East, folk music has always provided the core of the great classical music allied to religion; individual composition is less important than imaginative re-creation within a living tradition. In the West, however, we have had an erroneous culturally elitist viewpoint hammered into us by our biased and ignorant education system. We have been taught, quite wrongly, that 'art' music is vastly superior to 'folk' music.

During the musical revolution of the early twentieth-century a number of European and American composers turned to national folk music as a revivifying source for their individual creativity. By doing so, they reinstated the connection between the virtually moribund stereotype of 'art music' and the wellspring of a communal musical consciousness. Such recognition of folk music is not, however, identical to the life process of an enduring tradition; it is a specific cultural and artistic phenomenon.[3]

Environmental music forms a vast foundation for musical creation and composition, it is the group musical expression of many generations within their native land. So protean is this shared musical consciousness, that individuals return to it frequently for inspiration, example and even revelation.

3. *Individual*

Out of the environmental and cultural matrices, individual creators eventually crystallize. During the earliest stages, such as those of the ancient Greek civilization, the individuality is contained within the cultural matrix; this pattern is found widespread as late as the medieval period in Europe, and persists in oral (folk) traditions to the present day. In other words no *personalized* directions or notations define any particular unit of music in composition. The music is distinctive, strong, individual, but essentially co-operative and anonymous.[4]

It is this very co-operative quality which often frustrates modern interpreters of early music, even of periods as late as the Renaissance. Such music, though often individually composed, formed part of an organic social and musical tradition with its roots in oral transmission. Some of the most frustrating yet truly great works of early music can only be grasped in the light of oral traditions, and in a few rare cases in the context of specific magical or symbolic traditions embedded within traditional teachings, both orthodox religious and highly unorthodox.[5]

4. *Classical*

Our last stage is the classical period of eighteenth- and nineteenth-century European music, and this extends into the twentieth century. Although long-standing intellectual traditions are apparent in formal art music, it nevertheless degenerates into a rigid set of entities frozen upon paper by the notation system. The traditions become traditions of style, even of pretension, rather than areas of shared consciousness and experience.

Once this fourth phase begins to collapse, we experience the difficult and chaotic ferment of formalism in decay. Both modern serious music and modern popular music exhibit revolutionary attitudes, but both are heavily controlled and conditioned by increasing commercial pressures. Mass media has rapidly turned music into an industry rather than an art of communication.

As we are discussing musical metaphysics or the alchemy of music and changing consciousness, we must deliberately sidestep the standard historical approach to musical development. There is no suggestion that the Four Ages of Music and Consciousness replace or improve upon more detailed and comprehensive theories or works on musical history. They are merely a simple indicator of phases of progression, which also exist simultaneously as seeds in each cultural period.

Each of our four general stages of development (see Fig. 1) has one vital aspect in common: *they all employ natural sequences of sound emitted from physical sources.* The sources include the human voice, and the wide range of physically selective and controlled musical instruments. This may seem like a rather obvious and superficial statement, but it reaches to the root of metaphysical or magical music, and demands very careful consideration.

If we define the late twentieth century separately, it gives us a Fifth Age, still in transition or formation, that of the electronic musical source. The development of electronics in music, a synthetic control system for sound waves, is something startlingly new in application; the deeper implications are often missed or ignored by the composer or musician. Most electronic music is still, sadly, in the toy or gimmick stage (1987), but the speed with which equipment progresses far outstrips the human use and creative application.

The analogue synthesizers and digital computers which are widely used in popular and modern serious music do not genuinely reproduce or synthesize actual physical notes of music as created by natural instruments or the human voice. Sound synthesis cannot, in fact, re-create the sequences found in nature, which are sequences of extreme complexity and variation.

Musical scales are sequences of ascending and descending selected pitch (high and low notes in order). Due to a theory of *tempering* or compromise developed for keyboard tuning, a number of the natural intervals or distances and differences between high and low notes are intentionally corrupted or altered. We shall return to this tempering compromise in a later chapter, but for the present it is enough to say that it has disastrous effects when combined with the mathematical theories used in electronic instrument design. [6]

In synthesizers, particularly digital sampling machines in which sounds are programmed and reproduced upon the standard keyboard as music, a series of scales, intervals and overtones is generated. These are totally accurate in theory, and look fine upon the graph or drawing board, but they sound quite artificial. They are, literally, like nothing in nature.

As a professional composer I have worked with some very advanced digital computer instruments. These appear to be labour-saving and glamorous, and are acoustically intriguing, but they are surprisingly unversatile if we seek to go beyond the fashionable boundaries of sound synthesis. They cannot, in fact, synthesize a natural musical instrument with any genuine degree of success. The factors present in a natural wind or string instrument, or in the human voice, are profoundly complex, and the amount of hardware, software and special programming necessary even to approach such complexity is daunting. More to the point, the setting up and operational time is horribly long, and we can be in the ludicrous position of being surrounded by cubic volumes of refined instrumentation worth hundreds of thousands of pounds or dollars, and all merely to make a sound that can be perfectly produced from a simple stringed instrument or blown reed.

The use of such synthesizers in modern and especially commercial music is a clear reflection of our culture; we reject the natural and replace it by the intensely artificial. During the heyday of classical composition this rejection was a matter of *creative* formalism; today it has fully manifested in *expression* as physical synthesis, replacing organic sound sources with electronic sound generation. The human rejection of nature has moved from the creative realm into the expressive. We may see this process clearly shown in Fig. 2, a traditional metaphysical chart of the Four Worlds or phases of devolution from spirit to matter. Far from being an outmoded redundant conceptual model, this diagram has a direct relevance to cultural patterns, psychological mapping, physical growth,

Fig. 1 The Four Ages of Music

The Four Ages Model appears strongly in the pattern of Western culture, but Western culture has a powerful effect worldwide. The Four Ages are not limited to Western cultural history in isolation, but reflect a pattern of consciousness that appears collectively and individually throughout humankind. Cultures are still found today in the Primal and Environmental 'ages' of music, while it has been the growth of Western culture that has propelled the world at large into the present transitional (Fifth) period of chaotic ferment.

Although the Four Ages appear in historical linear time, this serial aspect is underpinned by each 'Age' being present in potential or seed form during any apparent era. Like the Four Elements, no Age exists solely without a relative foundation from the other three; thus if we analysed any culture in detail we would find aspects of primal, individual, environmental and art music, regardless of the predominant 'Age'.

Elements or Ages	Individuality	Cultural period
Primal music	the voice	primitive/prehistoric
Environmental music	expression through shared music/song	oral traditions of enduring time scale.

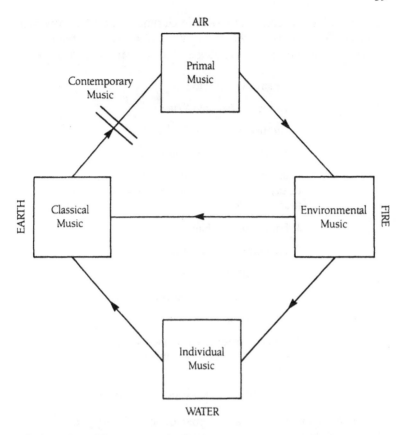

Elements or Ages	Individuality	Cultural period
Individual music	individual creativity distils out of the collective traditions	late medieval period onwards to 18th-19th centuries
Classical music	isolated individual formal/art composition now totally *written*	formal rigid and elitist period. 19th-20th centuries.
Contemporary music	individual seeking new music within/ beyond decaying formalism. Massive popular music, experiments with new instruments.	collapse of cultures. 20th-21st centuries.

40

and in our present context, musical development through history. More esoterically, it represents the basic pattern of origination, both for the individual psychic/body complex and for the material Universe.

> 1. Originative/Air into Fire
>
> 2. Formative/Fire into Water
>
> 3. Creative/Water into Earth
>
> 4. Expressive/Earth into new cycle.
>
> Traditional progression through Four Worlds or stages of manifestation. This is shown in music as follows:
>
> 1. Primal/Air into Fire
>
> 2. Environmental/Fire into Water
>
> 3. Individual/Water into Earth
>
> 4. Classical/Earth into new cycle
>
> (5. Modern/Transitional)
>
> The Stages merge together gradually and are not separated from one another by rigid boundaries.

Fig. 2 The Four Worlds of Manifestation

The Four Ages of Music and Consciousness in Application

To discover the principles behind music, those seemingly secret patterns that change our consciousness, we must first progress through the Four Ages and five stages listed above. As the fifth stage is our present crucial transitional era, we may see it as the exchange point between the ending of the Fourth Age (classicism) and the beginning of a new cycle.

If we follow the simple division of the Ages, bearing in mind always that they overlap and inter-relate in many complex ways (see Fig. 2) we can build up a tale of cultural evolution and regression expressed through musical development from the prehistoric period to the present day.

Before embarking upon this tale, which can only be told in the briefest manner in a short book, there is a central law of analogy that must be considered. *The stages of cultural development (expressed in instrumental and vocal music) are directly analogous to the creative or magical stages of music used for changing the individual consciousness.*

A primal musical concept is one that was *socially* expressed in the distant. or prehistoric past; a concrete realization of this concept in the present day can be achieved within the individual. It is essential that we do not confuse the primal patterns of the collective past with the seeds of consciousness that caused them to be expressed in their own time and place. Such seeds still exist within us today, in our own consciousness, ready to transform the present if they are aroused and correctly brought to fruition.

In other words, we may demonstrate certain primal magical or metaphysical musical laws by reference to prehistoric people, or to the Greeks or Celts, to the Hermetic musicians of the late medieval and Renaissance periods, but we do not have to copy or mimic their way of life. We bring such musical and magical changes through ourselves in the present, not through aping the selves of the historic past.

In each culture the musical seeds, the primal keys of changing consciousness and shaped sound (metaphysical music) manifest according to the lines of least resistance in that culture. The broadest line or channel is that of the communal imagination, expressed as folk and national music; this has been replaced and usurped to a large extent by product music issued through commercial enterprises and the media.

Behind or within this musical outlet of shared consciousness lies our set of patterns, the concentrated sequences by which music represents and re-creates changes of consciousness. In each century there are a few specific studies made of the magical effects of music, and there are still many active schools that employ musical systems for changing consciousness — including, of course, the orthodox churches. Within such practices there exists a core of metaphysics and metapsychology that reaches back into the depths of time, for its simple laws and practices are in fact timeless.[7]

Music and Changing Consciousness Today

A number of key patterns or systems remain surprisingly constant, and are still broadly disseminated as oral musical traditions. Such traditions take two main forms of expression, though these are interlinked in many fascinating ways.

The first is Eastern 'classical' or formal music, in which specific artistic and religious traditions are embodied in known and fairly rigid forms. Such forms are not rigid in the European sense of individual composition and notation, but act as strict matrices for the unfolding of a related tale, drama or ritual, or become in themselves a formalized religious rite.

The second is the folk music of both East and West, in which a protean body of music and song is stored and re-created in a shared consciousness. This consciousness emerges with distinctive racial and regional overtones, but oral music worldwide has certain shared characteristics. In the East, folk music is inextricably linked to formal or classical music, while in the West there is little connection other than through the work of specific composers.

If we examine these two routes of music, expressed through a group or racial consciousness, we can see that the first (formalized orthodox tradition or 'classicism') has a continual tendency towards degeneration, to devolution and ossification. This tendency is most apparent in European music, and has caused numerous musical revolutions.

In the West, music is held together by materialism, either that of patron groups or of commercial interests, while the East still retains a strong religious coherence, enabling the formal musical traditions to survive very long periods of time. Our second route for music through shared consciousness (oral or folk traditions) has a tendency to become static and ultra-conservative if it is divorced from the mainstream of the general culture. This is precisely the situation in the West today, where a remarkable body of song and music, once shared by many, is now rapidly disappearing in its genuine form. [8]

We can see this element of destruction very clearly indeed in the development of popular music in the West from folk music. Between the 1950s and the 1980s, basic musical patterns deriving from minority music in America have swept the world consciousness overboard. Through the ruthless exploitation of mass media, popular music has become a tool of manipulation on a very large scale.

From basic folk-blues, rock and roll developed. This in turn became 'rock' by the 1960s, and rapidly turned into the hybrid modern 'pop'. It is interesting to compare the modern product to its relatively recent folkloric source. Within two generations the quality of music and lyrics has degenerated, other than in the case of exceptional individual writers. Also greatly devolved is the technique, and the social validity of the material itself. Popular music no longer expresses the voice of the people — unless we accept that the people merely require trivia and banality.

While certain individual creative talents stand out in the popular field, the emphasis in the late twentieth century is upon *visual presentation*. Musical ability and creativity run as very poor seconds or thirds in the order of priority. Many famous recording artists and stage performers are genuinely unable to sing or play any musical instruments; they mime to pre-recorded tapes made by professional musicians, or generated in the electronic workshop of the recording studio. This bizarre tendency is now regarded as normal, reflecting the pressure to escape into artificial and synthetic realms of fantasy. These realms are sculpted for the profit of a tiny minority at the expense of the majority. Nor is the profit and expense merely monetary; its real power lies in the reduction of the communal imagination to a unified and trivial set of stereotypes.

Curiously, we shall find this same musical and psychological situation expressed in the historic past, in the liturgy of the orthodox churches. The essential difference, however, is that the Church based its use of sonic or magical keys upon a spiritual foundation, taken directly from the profound musical metaphysics of the ancients, and combined with the magical-religious uses of the common folk traditions.[9] No matter how redundant a formal religion becomes, it can still hold that seed of inner truth somewhere in its heart. Yet we cannot say as much of popular commercial music, which is the image-building religion of our present society.

It might seem from the foregoing pages that a case is being set out for reversion, for sneaking back into the cultural ambience of a romantic past. This is not intended, and we should not fall into the analogical trap (mentioned above) in which the seed concepts of one of our theoretical Four Ages are confused with the social or cultural forms through which they appeared in history.

Far from suggesting that we try to flee into an illusory and non-existent 'past', we should use our applied music to bring ourselves fully into the present. The present is the ultimate source of all being, from which the first Sound of Creation is uttered constantly. If we try to bring our consciousness alive through music, it must be music that reflects eternal presence. Neither the romantic past nor the materialist pseudo-future are sufficient.

3.

Primal Music —
Music and Originative Power

Originative music, which is equivalent to primal music in both human consciousness and society is *physical* and *metaphysical*, biological and psychological, material and spiritual. It is rooted in the unknown, yet utters forth its presence into the material world as sonic vibration. It also has the remarkable property of rearousing the unknown, the mysterious, within the consciousness of the listener.

This presence of music in two worlds, the physical and the metaphysical, is an essential feature of our musical growth both collectively and individually. Yet it has disappeared in quite recent times, leaving music wholly in the realm of the material world, which is to say, the erroneous concept of a world-view bounded solely and rigidly by materialist fantasies. At one extreme this imbalanced world-view generates the excesses of modern serious music, while at the other it allows the blatant commercialism of popular product.

The ancient metaphysicians and magicians repeatedly taught that the actual physical emission of sound, particularly of selected frequencies and patterns (music) was a reflection of an inner spiritual reality.[1] This inner reality has the potency of transformation, both personal and impersonal. If we are to use music today to change our consciousness, we must first rediscover this primal quality, and then apply it within ourselves. As it has a physical expression, it may be transferred directly from consciousness to consciousness without lengthy interfaces of meditational symbolism or religious ceremony. The magician not only uses music to prove the existence of altered states of awareness, of other dimensions and worlds, but also embeds this knowledge in musical sound, transferring it to whoever may listen.

Listening, hearing and comprehending are related but different processes, and although we may hear, or even listen to magical elements of music, we do not necessarily recognize or comprehend them. In a crude sense we find this stated in the music of television commercials and pop-songs, where the actual banality has a soporific or stimulating effect upon our stereotypes of imagination. The difference between conscious and unconscious listening runs far deeper than mere intellectual dissection.

One of the aims of our study of music and changing consciousness is to reveal exactly what our ears are hearing, to bridge the consciousness-gap between inner and outer music, between expression and imagination — and most important of all between the energies inherent in musical patterns and the corresponding but isolated energies of our combined psychic and physical expressions.

Why is music so magical? Why are the most profound spiritual revelations and modes of consciousness achieved traditionally through chant, while emitting and receiving certain musical patterns? The ancient and enduring answer is that music is an echo of the original impulse of divine creation.

Superficially this may appear to be a very orthodox and old-fashioned statement, yet our modern physicists have postulated several creation theories which are hardly different from the concept of Primal Breath or Creative Word found in magical, metaphysical and religious beliefs the world over. Our present thesis, however, is not an orthodox religious one, and the musical/psychological argument is not going to lead to any specific religious cult, church or practice. It deals with mystical and vital themes that underpin all religions, all creative discoveries about reality, and all aspects of consciousness.

The key word 'spirit' is derived from the concept of breath, and *inspiration* is still used as a direct reference to an influx of energy from some mysterious unknown source.[2] Musical inspiration may be creative or receptive, active or passive. We may be inspired to make a piece of music, or be inspired by the same work. The medium for transfer between these two poles, (active and passive or creative and receptive) is the element of Air, through which our sound waves or musical patterns travel from source to ear.

In metaphysical or alchemical music, the outer physical air, acting as communicative transferring medium for vibrations, is the expression of a more subtle Air, and of that same originative Spirit that breathed forth All from the Void.

On a human level, concepts or images are encapsulated in musical form and freely transferred from person to person; this process rapidly solidifies as sets of formulae. The most obvious example of this is the notation system, in which a musical work is frozen, but the solidification into standard formulae applies on a creative as well as an expressive level.

Metaphysically this rigidification corresponds to the First Breath uttering *Words* from the Void; these rapidly become crystallized as *Worlds* or orders of manifestation.

Before proceeding further, we should consider this set of concepts as an analogy to consciousness in the modern sense, for there is a wide gap between the ancient unified field or interlinked resonance of worlds and the theory of the individual psyche struggling for survival.

In the ancient philosophy, retained or sometimes hidden within the alchemical and Hermetic writings, there was an affirmed connection between human consciousness and the greater consciousness of the created world or Worlds. When the Renaissance theosophists revitalized and rewrote their inheritance of classical pagan lore, they applied it as a corrective to the separative and threatening world-view of the orthodox religion — the image of souls trapped in the clear-cut choice between heaven and hell, with the world of nature as a snare and delusion leading towards sin. Today we may use those same early philosophies as a corrective against rampant materialism, the concept of the evolutionary struggle and the embattled psyche lost in a wilderness of unconnected and hostile series of events.

Reductionism prevails not only in modern psychology, but as a long-term pattern of human deprivation; from the pan-spermic or unified archetypical consciousness of early pagan cultures we reduced our world-view to a duality with Christianity (God or the devil, heaven or hell); while with atheistic materialism we reduced it to a single meaningless and isolated consciousness.

This pattern of reduction is found in music, and underpins and corrects our customary historical image of the so-called evolution of musical consciousness. From the primal and early cultures, in which music was a collective and holistic response to intimations of a shared consciousness, a unified and dreamlike music arose. We can still find this music, to a certain extent, in the great oriental classical music, and in the fragments of genuine Western folk music.

The formal religion of Christianity had a profound effect upon European music; this effect was not only one of musical technical application as is often asserted, for the general music of the people was applied to the liturgy of the Church, and not vice versa.[3] The effect was upon the consciousness of many generations, and led directly to the development of aspects of music which are reflected in society today as capitalism and materialism.

To be more specific, the authoritarian and dualistic struggle (God and the devil, faith and heresy, free will and divine ordination) created the formal music of Europe. Passing through a series of developments in which liturgical and individual music seemed to separate from one another, we nevertheless arrived at a position where the so-called classical music of Europe appeared. This music, containing many wonderful and transcendent achievements, was founded upon the old duality; it was the music of a selective socially priviledged elite from which the majority of society were excluded. It was the music of male stereotypical dominance, confined to a rigid conventional system of composition, performance and notation.

When the religious authority was finally exploded, the stereotype passed into the hands of science, creating the isolated individual adrift in a meaningless (but scientifically provable) world. We find the lure of heaven in a material sense, with the illusions of achievement or success, or merely as possessions, but this is an individual isolated heaven, without any deeper or collective value.

In music we have experienced a series of revolutions both in avant-garde serious work and in popular music disseminated through advancing technology. The drift in the common consciousness is towards increasing fragmentation and isolation; this process is most clearly found in product music, where short ritualized fragments of melody and rhythym are accompanied by ephemeral dramatic images (the video) in which each purchaser may identify something of his or her self for a few minutes. Within a short time, this musical stereotype is replaced with another product item, and so on.

The potential for unifying these fragments is present but is seldom realized, for a variety of reasons financial, political, and the more subtle problem that the industry itself is entrapped in the illusion system despite its own cynicism and crude psychology of purchaser manipulation.

This modern situation is clearly similar to that of the primal musical world, but with a number of extremely important differences. In both cases we have images shared by large numbers of people, and music held within a common consciousness. But the first, primal music, was rooted in deeply regenerative sets of relationship to nature, to images of gods and goddesses, and to an overall shared consciousness which was unable to make a division between the inner and outer worlds. The medium of that sharing was the collective psyche and a powerful group memory expressed as music, poetry, dance and song.

In our modern popular culture the music is rooted in an intentionally ephemeral set of relationships to an ever-changing pursuit of novelty, to images of popular performers, and to an overall consciousness utterly directed to the outer world and its fashions. The medium of sharing is an individual distribution of technology, in which the memory is replaced by electronic storage and retrieval systems which externalize attention and repeatedly dissolve any development of continual creative shared consciousness.

This comparison may also be extended to modern serious music, which operates to a smaller social group, but tends towards similar practices (the increasingly high technology of music reproduction, the star performer syndrome, the growth of highly isolated and inaccessible music — this last being one intellectually significant difference between serious and popular music).

When the ancient models of Breath, Word and Worlds are used in our argument, they need not be taken as religious or mysterious terms; they are an alternative set of concepts which enable us rapidly to summarize and encapsulate lengthy comparisons such as the paragraphs above. The degeneration or devolution of music and social expression, the polarization of opposites, and the ultimate externalization which is close to primal origination (all the musical and social phases briefly summarized) are expressed quite clearly upon a map or glyph popularly known as *The Tree of Life*. Far from being a superstitious tool or the incomprehensible mystery of the elitist occult fraternity, the Tree of Life is a flexible and quite accessible model which helps and enables our understanding of music and changing consciousness.

As the Tree of Life will be used repeatedly in our main argument, and forms the foundation for the polarity patterns that arise out of the consciousness (within the system of analysis employed here to relate music to the human psyche), a short summary and definition is essential at this stage. I would like to stress that any reader wishing to apply the musical, psychological, magical or therapeutic methods demonstrated, or the exercises in our later chapters should study the Tree of Life description and diagrams. Furthermore, the published material on the Tree of Life is often contradictory, confusing and sectarian; the reader already familiar with one or other of the variants, even the experienced meditator or practitioner with the Tree symbolism, should not be tempted to pass over the restatements offered here, as they provide clear keys to the present system without claiming to replace or dispute other uses of the glyph (which is universal and open-ended, and therefore open to infinite application and variation).

The Tree of Life
During the medieval period in Europe, a symbolic structure appeared

in illustrated form, based upon the male/female positive/negative polarities. This illustration is known today as the Qabalistic Tree of Life, and it has played an important role in metaphysical and magical literature and practice in the West for several centuries.

Although the Tree of Life is generally said to be Hebrew in origin, this assumption is no longer valid. The Tree came into early literature by way of Jewish mystical tradition in Europe, but it merged with a native Tree of Life (non-mathematical in presentation). Both variants are significant but non-exclusive representations of a widespread glyph or map of polarities. The polarities shown are identified with both human consciousness and physical expression (the microcosm) and with solar or stellar creation and manifestation (the macrocosm).[4]

These same laws of polarity and proportion were also known to the ancient Greeks; we know them today in the form of the Platonic solids, a set of conceptual models, and through the teachings traditionally ascribed to Pythagoras, who employed music as a proof of universal laws.[5] The modern Tree of Life owes as much to classical sources as it does to native Celtic and Near-Eastern mysticism or astrology.

We shall be using this symbolic key, the Tree of Life, in several ways and forms during our analysis of music; not because it is a religious or superstitious emblem, but for its extreme expressive subtlety. It acts as a master map to show relationships and concepts which become cumbersome in word form. It has been employed by many writers and teachers, ranging through obscure works on ritual magic, alchemical texts, Jesuit musical treatises, and more recently in popular textbooks on psychology.[6]

Fig. 3 will be helpful in relating to our main text, and will repay careful study and thought.

A detailed knowledge of the multitude of correspondences hung upon the Tree of Life in literature is not required. We can follow the musical arguments by relating to the shape and the implied relationships between the poles or stations of the Tree of Life very easily and simply. Many of the correspondences found in literature are inaccurate and redundant, and some versions are deliberately confused to bewilder the student.[7]

Sphere	Simple Attributes
1. The Crown	Universal point of Origin, First Breath.
2. Wisdom	Word of Power, the exploding stars.
3. Understanding	Space, the Mother Deep.
4. Mercy	Energies of 'Giving' or construction.
5. Severity	Energies of 'Taking' or negation.

6.	Beauty	Balance, energies in a state of Harmony.
7.	Victory	Energies polarizing as modes of consciousness (emotions).
8.	Honour or Glory	Energies polarizing as modes of consciousness (intellect).
9.	Foundation	Biological matrix of energies.
10.	Kingdom	Expression of all combined energies as outer collective world (psychological, biological, material).

The Tree of Life is made up of three pillars or polarities:

Middle: Neutral/Balancing
Left: Catalytic/Receptive
Right: Analytic/Active

Each Pillar polarizes the flow of interacting Spheres or Qualities of Being. Each Sphere has a specific polarity which is reflected in the human elemental psyche. Traditionally each Sphere is associated with a planet.

All Ten spheres are connected by paths in a polarity or 'circuit' diagram which shows both cosmic and individual configurations in a flat symbol accessible to the human mind.

Sphere	Polarity	Quality	Planet
One	Origination (pre-polarity)	Origination	(Uranus)
Two	Male	Wisdom	Neptune
Three	Female	Understanding	Saturn
Four	Male 2	Mercy	Jupiter
Five	Female 2	Severity	Mars
Six	Balanced (Male/Female)	Beauty	Sun
Seven	Female 3	Victory	Venus
Eight	Male 3	Glory/Honour	Mercury
Nine	Resolving (balanced)	Foundation	Moon
Ten	Expression of all Spheres	Kingdom	Earth

The Abyss is the rift or gap between Originative consciousness and the remainder of the Tree of Life, symbolized by the planet Pluto.

Classical Planetary attributions are sadly confusing for the general reader; their polarity reflects cultural symbols taken out of context, with male figures (Saturn, Mars) replacing two essential female figures upon the Tree of Life.

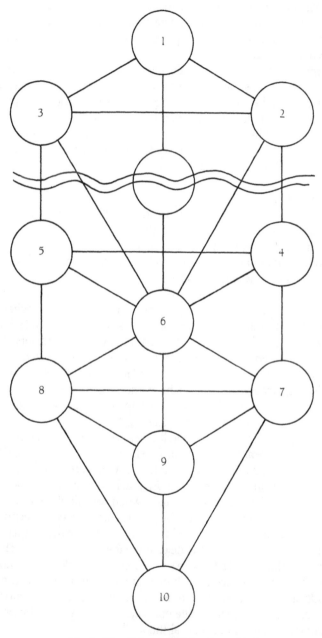

Fig. 3 The Polarities of the Tree of Life

The Paths upon the Tree of Life form psychic or sacro-magical images and symbols which depict the interactions between the sets of Spheres. These are not included in our present summary, but are traditionally shown as the Tarot Trumps.

In musical symbolism the Paths represent combination-tones (when musical notes are struck together to create interactive frequencies) and also represent the *approach* or quality of utterance of each metaphysical tone or pitch. Most Spheres may be *approached* from at least three directions or Paths; in music or vocal tones these would be three *qualities of utterance*, conditioned by the consciousness of the pair of Spheres linking the Path concerned.

Primal Music
Primal Music comes directly from the Breath of Life. In the human organism this breath gives birth to the voice. The voice is our primal instrument for communication, emotion, inspiration, verbal units of meaning, and for musical shapes made from ascending and descending levels of pitch (the musical scales).

When we hear certain unusual types of song or chant, such as a Bhuddist mantram, an Islamic prayer call or a Christian plainchant, we are receiving primal music in varying degrees of complexity and structure. In the West, the plainchant could be replaced by an oral traditional ballad or song; both represent the remaining expressions of a Western magical chant system which is usually presumed to be non-existent or lost. Not all folksong, however, comes into this magical chant category, but a certain proportion does, and the highly developed formal plainchant of the Church was partly drawn from folksong.[8]

It is only too easy for reader and listener to confuse primal music with barbaric or ignorant and boorish music. Modern product recordings are quite 'primitive' in comparison to the remarkable subtleties heard on genuine field recordings of traditional and primal music. Even 'primitive' is a dangerous relative term when we talk of music or other cultural activities, for quite primitive people without modern technology or medicine can and have produced music of remarkable quality.

The subtleties displayed by the chant of the Aka pygmies, or Tibetan Tantric monks, or the Hebridean solo singer, are not matters of contrived style.[9] They are the direct result of attuning to an inner music, to the sounds of nature. These inner musical sounds can be approached and discovered in a number of different ways, and are proven by rational scientific analysis and acoustical theory.[10]

When we talk of the sounds of nature, we must include not only the exterior phenomenal world, but the human body-psychic complexity. The natural laws which are found within music apply physically to both the human body and to other expressions within the natural world, and they have quite notable biological and psychological effects. Although we are dealing with primal music as vocal music, there are some instrumental techniques or non-techniques which aim to mirror nature, and thus express the Unknown beyond and within nature. One of the increasingly popular examples of such music in the West is the shakuhachi, a Zen Buddhist flute. In its native environment, this instrument is used not to play music, but to generate the inspired (breath created) sounds of divine nature. With metaphysical correspondences for each tone and each finger-hole, the shakuhachi is a musical Tree of Life.

Although we have given an oriental example, the same principles are found in the basic musical traditions of the West, though they are often clouded or confused. Any musical instrument, as we shall discover, is a clear representation of the metaphysical and physical polarity relationships shown upon the Tree of Life. Differences lie only in the consciousness that is expressed by the player through the instrument, yet the magical sounds remain no matter what is being played.

The relationship between the human voice, breath, sound, musical shape or contour, is not a contrivance; it is a property of physics. We shall return to this important concept several times, particularly in the context of ancient and Hermetic or alchemical music, and in our practical work on magical/psychological chanting.

The Voice, the Instrument and the Creative Word

At this point, we can draw some basic comparisons between the human voice, musical instruments, and the metaphysics of creation, as stated through inward cognition and intuition. Although this is not a scientific textbook, it is worth suggesting that there are many parallels between the ancient metaphysical models and modern physics. Metaphysics, however, is proven by experience of new levels of awareness, and not by comparison to materialist theories or practices.

The value of music is that it links the physical and metaphysical together in the human consciousness, creating modes of awareness in which the creative unity of all being is glimpsed, albeit briefly. With specific magical or transformative music, we can extend those moments of heightened perception; with constant work it is even possible to bring the transformative element right through into the physical body. This physical effect is immediately apparent in terms of actual sonic vibration and sympathetic resonance within our physical entity, but it runs through the interaction between the inner and outer being, the psyche and the biological expression of the psyche. We shall return to this theme repeatedly as we progress.

To come to grips with the basic concepts, we must employ some basic metaphysical vocabulary. This is not used in an orthodox religious sense (though the meaning would be similar if it was), for pure metaphysics is obscured by dogma or cult conditioning.

The use of *primal imagery* corresponds to the use of *primal sound* in music, and both work as concentrated sources or seeds for more lengthy expositions in either art or science. The basic terms are used here in the form of a concentrated set of reference points for concepts which must be absorbed in meditation. They are not merely words to be read and skipped over. In applying the primal vocabulary we are following traditional usage that extends worldwide and is hallowed by thousands of years of practice. Many different languages employ this basic terminology, but we shall express it always in simple terms.

The Original Word was uttered with the First Breath. The Word is the power exhaled by the mysterious source or Spirit. In physics it is known as the 'origin of the universe', while in metaphysics it is known as the 'origin of the Worlds'. We may approach this concept materially through science, or poetically through intuition. Both devolve into a type of religion or dogma quite rapidly, but devolution is inherent in the origin of the Worlds.

A very simple mathematical relationship has always been employed to demonstrate our inward cognition of reality. In this system, the relationships between the numbers 1-4 plays a central role. The Word manifests through Four Worlds, while its cycle of rotation exhibits Four phases, phases which later appear as the Four Elements. This basic theme is shown in our diagrams in Chapter 5.

From the Fourfold pattern, a Tenfold set of relationships develops, with polarities of male/female, positive/negative, active/receptive inherent in its flow of energy. The Tree of Life demonstrates this set of relationships, as does the Pythagorean Tetractys, shown in Fig. 4. The basis for this development lies in the numerical fact that $1+2+3+4=10$, a superficially simplistic statement, but one with many mathematical and conceptual ramifications.

When a human utters a word or musical note, this initially metaphysical process immediately reflects itself in the acoustic physical event of utterance. The breath triggers the vocal chords, and controlled by will or inspiration, certain defined frequencies are generated in the air and in the cavities of the body, particularly those of the skull.

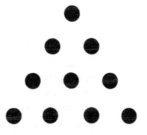

Fig. 4 The Tetractys

To the materialist psychologist, the metaphysics is merely a fanciful theory that is grounded in the biological act of vocal utterance. To the magician or meta-psychologist, the biological and physical acoustic act is merely a reflection of an utterance that runs through all existence.

All being, all life, all utterances from birdsong to vast exploding galaxies of stars — all are breathed forth by an unknown source. This harmonic relationship is reflected in the human voice, for although we think that we are singing one single note, such is certainly not the case. In any one single note there is a series of related but mainly unheard elements or 'other notes.' These are technically known as *partials, overtones,* or *harmonics.* We may not all be able to hear these partials, but if we could freeze our vocal note and dissect it, we would find them to have a mathematical relationship. This can be done in a variety of simple experiments, and is clearly outlined in many basic studies of acoustics and music.[11]

When we examine the partials, we find that they have a mathematical and proportional relationship very similar to that shown in the magical or metaphysical models used by the ancients. These models, such as the Tetractys or the Tree of Life, analogized both human consciousness and biological structure, and related them to Divine consciousness and universal structure. They were *harmonics* of one another, the macrocosm and the microcosm.[12]

In certain primal music, the inspired singer can actually render harmonics that are audible to the listener, giving the curious effect of singing two notes or more at once. The additional notes are the partials or harmonics that are always present, but they are given emphasis and amplification by special techniques. This has an obvious analogy with the inner techniques of meditation or visualization that are employed and amplified by the act of chanting; the previously hidden but ever-present aspects of consciousness are brought into the outer perception, transforming previous false assumptions about apparent reality.

There is a famous recording of Tibetan monks singing at a pitch extremely low for the human voice, while simultaneously chanting a pattern of higher notes and tones. This recording demonstrates the technique in a most startling and dramatic manner, and often has peculiar physical effects upon the listener.[13] In the invocations and chants of priests, monks, shamans or medicine men, the upper partials, the haunting higher sounds that arise out of the basic notes, are used as evidence of a spiritual presence inherent in the material world. We may reasonably infer that similar techniques were widespread in both pagan and early Christian inspirational chant.

There is evidence from early Church authorities for magical or inspirational chanting, generally banned and discouraged for political reasons. The element of inspiration in religious chant was central to the pagan rituals,[14] and is still employed in many minority cults and magical groups today.

In European and American folk music, specific decorative vocal effects are heard, which rely upon natural partials. (These involve a sudden transfer to the *third* step of the scale, using a natural note which is rather different in pitch to that found on the keyboard equivalent. More rarely a note will be raised by an interval of one *fourth* or *fifth*. In both cases the new note is a partial or overtone rather than a deliberately sung step of the scale.)[15]

More rarely, a free use of partials and extra notes is found in European music, in inspired melismatic chanting. It occurs in the services or meetings of certain cults, both black and white, and has an origin that transcends cultural or racial background. Modern charismatic Christians and Pentacostalists can create a very remarkable musical entity, incorporating the range of harmonic relationships based upon natural overtones or partials, arising in an inspired manner rather than from written notes. Similar music can also be created by the individual composer, but only rarely with a natural quality.[16] Such chanting is a last vestige of communally inspired music in the West; similar music is still current in Africa, Asia and many Eastern countries. In all cases it is linked to a religious or magical practice.

One interesting aspect of the inspirational group chant is that it is very difficult to imitate or fake. During a technical analysis of a number of recordings, both commercial and situational, the author found that the commercial discs of charismatic cult chanting always employed pre-selected blocks of notes. In other words, they were written out or selected in advance. The situational or field recordings, made at events where genuine inspired chanting occurred, occasionally contained a remarkable web of interwoven vocal sounds; these were presumably the result of the group consciousness created by religious fervour.

We have dealt with several contemporary examples from Eastern and Western sources, as these give some suggestion of the vocal quality and power of primal music. The music used for meditation, magic, alchemy, metaphysics and spiritual practices worldwide can be very concentrated indeed, and far transcends the group chant of the modern religious cult. When examining this type of music, we must always remember that it can be found in two basic aspects: group inspiration, and specialist trained invocation. In the ancient Mysteries both elements worked together; today the first (group inspiration) is random and rare, while the second (trained invocation) is almost nonexistent other than in a few monasteries in both the East and the West.

Primal music, therefore, is a physical sound pattern within which other sound patterns are inherent. It corresponds to the relationships employed by metaphysicians (both Christian and non-Christian) to provide maps of Creation, of the inner worlds, and of the human entity. It also works as a powerful medium for the transfer of consciousness, enabled by the element of Air. This Air may be the physical gas or atmosphere, or may be a more subtle pervasive air, that which the unknown breathed forth to utter the Word of Beginnings.

Particular emphasis is given to primal music in this study, simply because it is the least understood aspect of our musical consciousness. To render the psychological, meditational or magical exercises of the Elemental calls effectively, the student needs to have some real contact with primal music within his or her self. No one assumes that a mere intellectual description will create such a contact, but it provides a few basic reference points for the imagination, which act as anchors during the early phases of musical metaphysics.

As shown in our schematic Fig. 1, the relationship between the four aspects of music (primal, environmental, individual, classical or formal) is not merely a linear or pseudo-evolutionary progression; they may interact with one another in a direct manner. This interaction is most obviously found in the works of composers who both consciously and unconsciously have returned to primal or environmental musical roots for their inspiration or foundation.

In our own application of music as a psychic science, the elemental rotations or calls (see Chapter 5) are merely one simple example of a perpetual rotation and spiral that occurs in both consciousness and nature. We may, and often do, contact primal and potent roots through quite absurd sources — a phrase of a popular song, a passage in an otherwise unremarkable piece of art music. This diffuse and temporary arousal is insufficient for active rebalancing of the musically deprived psyche, and reflects our astonishing passivity and lack of direction in musical matters.

The musical shapes found in metaphysics are drawn from nature; they represent the human intellect analysing and formalizing an inspirational urge to musical expression. This is heard, obviously, in birdsong, and was enlivened for many thousands of years in the inspired jubilation or ululation of ethnic music. When the term 'ethnic music' is employed, we must use it in its proper sense of music natural to various peoples in their own environment; it does not mean commercial recorded music for minority consumer groups, though this may include some genuine ethnic music on occasion.

Primal Music Becomes Environmental Music
At the moment of utterance, the inspirational call becomes modified not only by the physical body, but by the collective or resonant influence of the environment. This generates the very distinctive style and subtlety of folk music or ethnic music worldwide. It is at this point in the growth of music, in its spiral progression, that we must pause. There is no need to take the historical or cultural aspects of the analysis further, for the later stages are well represented in many excellent books on musical history. More important is the fact that metaphysicians or religious and magical specialists (pagan and Christian alike) fully understood this bridging area in which inspired vocal utterances became stylized as regional or national music. Such patterns were specifically applied, modified or concentrated, to generate physical, psychic and spiritual responses in both the individual and the assembled group.[17]

The primal musical patterns were further vitalized by concentration and development of techniques which related to the inner and outer worlds, and certain basic chants achieved an organic growth and increase of potency by centuries of such applied consciousness. The most obvious examples of this potency, well known to the general listener, are the monastic chants of both East and West.[18]

If we are to avoid religious sectarianism, we must boil the material down to its basic constituents, the *prima materia* of the alchemist, and discover for ourselves the foundations and building blocks that underpin music and consciousness, both specific as in magical-religious chant and instrumental music, and general, as in music from art and popular sources.

4.

Acoustics, Music and the Musical Examples

The exercises and diagrams in the following chapters are made as basic and simple as possible, with the hope that they can be followed and applied by musicians and non-musicians alike. Indeed, they may be easier for the non-musician, as he or she has no musical preconceptions or specialized knowledge to confuse or sidetrack direct application and understanding.

In preparing the examples, a specific and important problem arises immediately, and this has a number of symbolic implications that are illuminating in the context of music and changing consciousness. The problem, which I have solved in the time-hallowed musical tradition of stating it while otherwise ignoring it, is that of *tempering*.

Tempering is a technical system of tuning or modification, which is applied worldwide in art and popular music, though it is less apparent in traditional music. The European system of *equal temperament* enables instruments to play together without certain clashes of 'tuning' or pitch, and is particularly important for the piano keyboard.

In nature musical pitch expands — which is to say that it makes a perpetual spiral of fifths in which there are few neat mathematical correspondences. In art, these expanding fractions, once used as evidence of the perpetual creation of existence, are clipped down to conform with keyboard application and with a unified musical theory. This practice, apparently useful in the solution of musical problems for ensemble playing, reflects our urge to find systems and logically controlled patterns in nature. The minute natural expansion (in which twelve fifth intervals should, but do not, equate with seven octaves) is doctored by clipping a small amount of each successive fifth until it comes into step with the range of seven octaves.[1]

The above paragraph is necessarily a simplification of the theory, and the reader who wishes to go into it in depth will find it in various reference works cited in the Bibliography.

In our visual context, in which octaves, scales and intervals, are shown upon a circular or spiralling ground, the expansive mathematics of the natural fifth are ignored, and the system of equal temperament is assumed.

The intervals concerned, and the differences that are subtracted for conformity cannot usually be heard to be at variance. In modern listeners pitch discretion is very poor indeed due to the conformity and limitation of the keyboard over the last two centuries.

But what does this musical underworld of unsuspected notes imply for our system of musical alchemy? Merely that the formal theories of music as taught or published are by no means as accurate as we have been led to believe. If we follow the natural implications and expressions of our voices, we are on the right track to refreshing our musical consciousness. There is no need, in other words, to worry about the 'in tuneness' of your vocal calls if you try singing the exercises which follow. More important, we do not need to strive to create logical all-inclusive musical theories that close up and restrict the magical or psychological implications into sets of 'correspondences' that must be adhered to come what may. This method leads us back into the dreary situation where certain notes are said to correspond to certain inner or metaphysical concepts, but hardly ever seem to make any practical connection.

Lest I be accused of being so general that the theories lose their power in a welter of kindly liberation, it is worth realizing that nature makes her own adjustments. The system of temperament is with us and is part of our collective musical consciousness; but for every element of unnatural device, there is a harmonic pattern which restates the natural resonances. These are well known in the mysterious sub-tones or combinations heard in bells, or in the skilful use of piano keyboard, creating sounds which do not, logically, exist in the original pitched notes. More directly, we can hear massively complex overtones in any orchestral work, and modern composers deliberately strive to create such resonances in despite of the limitations of the tuning and notation system that they are forced to work with. But this is not merely true of modern music, for the most staid of composers in the gross nineteenth-century traditions cannot avoid the resonances that occur in musical instruments. Only electronic music can do this — to our great detriment.[2]

It is in this natural realm of harmonics, overtones and interactive tones that music really operates. The musical alchemical formulae in the following chapter are based upon a series of overtones reduced to notes which may be approximated upon the piano keyboard for practical purposes. We are more concerned in psychological or magical music with *shape* than with *pitch*; it is the relativity demonstrated and enlivened by the music that has the inner or therapeutic effect, and not the isolation of any one specific note and its mathematical verification or flaw.

Pitch

It has been generally accepted in magical or metaphysical music that there are certain pitches, defined levels of vibration (rates per second) which correspond to or even stimulate power centres, moods, planetary functions within consciousness and so forth. For the sake of the general theory and ease of application, we will be using the standard scale of C major for our musical examples, but this is not intended as definitive, nor was it definitive when employed by earlier meta-musicians.

Our so-called standard pitch, generalized for international use, is quite a modern invention, and cannot have a true relationship to consciousness in nature. We only need to look at the instruments of preceding centuries to find preferences for lower (and sometimes higher) pitch standards. In early music, pitch was a matter of relativity and not of absolute definition. This intimate sense of relativity and shape persists in environmental or folk music throughout the world, achieving harmony and integration of intonation that seem remarkable to the trained musician, as no formality or science is involved.

Such a sense of pitch, of relationship, comes not from numerical theory or standardization, but from an inner quality of proportion, beauty and intuition. We find this intuition extended beyond musical notes, for in the great traditions there are similar holistic or harmonic relationships between music and words, and between music and dance. Folksong collectors often found that ballad singers were not able to separate the words and melody of their ancient songs, while those who could write or dictate words often assumed that through knowledge of the text, the collector would instantly know the melody.[3] This is not the simple rustic displaying his or her ignorance, but an expression of a very deep creative intuition, in which words, story, melody and performance all combined into one magical emission or sacred entity. In folksong this sacred quality is usually absent, but the magical quality is present in many examples.

The relationship between music and dance is likewise an intuitive one; to know the music is sufficient to know the dance, and vice versa. We find this supported by ancient evidence, including sources within the early Church.[4] While touring Brittany as a performer, I was taught a number of Breton dance tunes by villagers, and in most cases they insisted that as I knew the melody, I therefore knew the dance. Dance and music were an inseparable entity in ancient times, and this fusion still exists within ourselves today, revealed in ethnic practices, but concealed in the modern man or woman in the city by an overlay of conditioning.

The so-called problem of pitch should not be a problem at all. It is a matter of proportion and relativity, and not a rule of firmly defined vibrations per second. The firm definition is invaluable when it comes to certain types of standardized group music making, but it is only one possible pitch standard, and we lose certain biological responses and rhythms by its constant use. To prove this, listen to any old-style instrument in flat pitch; most people immediately comment upon the expressive quality, the subtlety, the refreshing or even surprising effect of the music. Then immediately hear the same piece of music played upon a modern piano, or even worse, upon a keyboard synthesizer.

The use of proportion to demonstrate metaphysical propositions has always been central to music, from the times of the Pythagorean Greeks to the present day. Certain proportions demonstrate the relationships between planetary orbits, and between the inner orbits or modes or consciousness of which the outer planets are merely physical analogies within the greater consciousness of the Solar System. There is no reason why we should not use our modern instruments or scales to express these intervals, proportions and relationships for practical purposes; providing we do not assume that there is any ultimate or unchanging value to their vibration rates. The tuning or selected number of vibrations per second is merely a slice from the spectrum of sound; it varies from culture to culture and from century to century. The proportions, the shapes, and the truly archetypical concepts and matrices implied by *music* have a quality that transcends and also underpins time, serial pitch, and serial limitations to the application of sound and human consciousness.

Using the Model

To gain the best advantage from the alchemical-musical experiment outlined in the following chapter, I would recommend the following:

1. Read the entire chapter through two or three times without attempting to correlate the visual symbols or experiment with the actual musical patterns described. Become accustomed to the progression of concepts of the Elemental system; it is an ancient and effective

conceptual model, but the modern reader needs to adjust to it slowly and naturally; it is a rhythmic and holistic model, not merely one of intellectual deliberation or satisfaction.

2. Once you are familiar with the material, begin to move from one diagram and its notes to the other, following the development as you progress.

3. Draw each diagram out, stage by stage, following the development of the concepts. This drawing need be no more than a mere sketch copied from the book, but if you know the value of each step, it is the most effective way of learning a metaphysical system, and replaces thousands of words. In magical teaching traditions, pupils are often set to draw such symbols before they are given any indication of the meaning, and even to meditate upon them. In the use of such methods, the inner or higher meaning breaks through into the intellect, illuminating it with an archetypical pattern — the very purpose and aim of metaphysical philosophy or magical psychology.

4. Return to the beginning of the experiment, and retrace it musically, step by step. This may be done upon a keyboard, but is more powerful vocally.

5. When you are familiar with the musical spirals, squares and calls, proceed to the practical exercises outlined in our later chapters, but not before. If you jump ahead and try out some of the exercises, they may well work for you; it is better to have such material in context, and to be familiar with its inner development. The basic growth of the calls, the Tree of Life, and the meditational or therapeutic exercises can only come alive if it is complete from roots (the early symbols and cycles) to crown, (the Tree of Life and power centres in the life-system of the singer).

5.

A Musical Looking Glass
or
Hermetic Speculum

The alchemists, from whom our subtitle has been borrowed,[1] were among the last of a long procession of thinkers, experimenters and philosophers who viewed music in a manner entirely different from that of today. Whereas modern culture certainly claims music as an art, at its best, or as a commercial product in its lowest form, our predecessors used it in a way which is often incomprehensible to the modern mind. It was accepted that music epitomized certain natural laws, not only of physics, but of the metaphysics from which physics was derived. This belief was not in any way limited to an 'emotional' or 'creative' application of music, but depended upon the premise that *physical emission of sound* was an outer and audible agency of an inner and transcendent power. The composition of music was irrelevant to this interpretation, as was personal artistic merit or 'originality', the very qualities prized so highly today. These qualities, arduously sought by the classical and modern composer or performer of music, from the most strenuously creative to the merely superficial, were only side-effects of the metaphysical medium of music as supposed by the Hermetic philosophers.

What was assigned great importance was pattern, and beyond pattern, meta-pattern, higher orders or modes of shape which expressed themselves through the lower order media of music. It is this lack of concern with personality in musical composition (as understood in the classical or popular sense) that permeates folk and traditional music the world over, and which frustrates transcription. Too often the assumption is made that early musical notation was inept, for only such inefficiency could account for the lack of rigidity and definition. This is far indeed from the truth.[2]

Natural folk music and early written music derived directly from oral musical systems, applied creativity in performance rather than inscription.

This is not entirely consonant with the modern concept of 'improvisation', for it worked through a process of re-creation from primary core melodies, rather than a fixation of personal creativity in writing, and was far from 'free' in the sense of lacking rules or discipline. The rules, however, were *implicit*, and were not confined to serial or structural forms as we understand music in the post-classical period of the twentieth century.

To the alchemical or Hermetic musicologists, who inherited their understanding from the written and oral traditions of ancient cultures, a corpus of traditionally defined melodies and scales was an example of the hallowed approach to music as a sacred science. The entire matter was taken beyond mere religion or cultism, however, for Hermetic students of music through the ages (from the semi-legendary Pythagoras to the modern Rudolph Steiner) all stated that regular musical expression was the result of a higher order of pattern. This higher order was implicit in ordinary music, but explicit in its own realm or state of being.

In other words, music worked because of a secret content which lay in the expression of sound, not necessarily connected to personal creativity other than by inevitable coincidence. This should not be confused with the scientific knowledge that certain acoustic frequencies or vibrations have specific effects upon the human listener, though such knowledge undoubtedly played a part in the expression and development of music as a sacred or magical vehicle of consciousness.

The apparently 'secret' content of music was not found through an examination or an abstraction of the laws of acoustics, but in the subtle perception of archetypes from which the laws of physical acoustics were said to have devolved. This is a very important concept indeed, and should not be overlooked when examining the Hermetic approach to music, as represented in both liturgical and literary examples. The ancient Greeks, as represented by the figure of Pythagoras, had discovered certain simple laws of proportion which apply to physical sound.[3] These laws were assumed to be automatic in the emission of sound, and were refined through limitation in the performance of any type of music. To put it more simply, any controlled or defined part of the broad spectrum of noise can become music — if it harmonizes with certain peculiar and often mysterious physiological rhythms and tonal aptitudes found in humankind.

In noise, all the harmonic sequences are mixed together in a very complex and apparently random manner, but in music, certain recognizable areas of those sequences are rendered prominent and relatively pure. That this purity is relative and partly subjective is well known to the modern acoustic physicist, and in this respect any Hermetic scholar would have agreed with the materialist findings — but from a different reasoning and a different basic conceptual model.

The ancients were so aware of the power of music that certain modes or rotations of a given scale of controlled intervals of pitch were deemed to be ravishingly powerful. Not only do we have evidence of this belief from the Greeks, but we also find it reccurring centuries later in Christian liturgical chant, and in the strict ruling by the Church authorities that banned certain scales or modes in worship. Not only were these modes dangerous, but one in particular was the regular vehicle for bawdy songs!

While the modern reader may find this attitude quaint or amusing on one hand, or redolent of suppressive propaganda on the other, it was clearly taken very seriously by those who adopted it, and is derived from ancient magical practice in the use of music for invocation of unseen powers. Such concern and precision over the mere use of a scale seems odd to the modern musician who expects his music to be tonally and modally defined before he ever plays or sings a note, but traditional and oral music is not confined in such a way, and the same melodic shape may be freely re-expressed in several different scales or modes. This flexibility was retained in early written music, and in various forms of non-standard musical writing or notation well into the nineteenth century, such as the dissenting worshipper's 'shape note' system freely used in the United States. [4]

It is worth repeating at this point that the flexibility concerned is not necessarily the product of ignorance, but is derived from a traditional musical model or system now virtually lost and forgotten. Evidence of this model is found scattered through folk musics, and many examples, such as the communication system for bagpipe music in the Highlands of Scotland, were wiped out by force of arms. Whatever this system may have been, the Scottish version practised as late as the eighteenth century enabled musicians to learn and retain a very large number of long and complicated works of music entirely without written notes. Irish harpers of the same period employed various mnemonic systems for composition and re-creation, and traditional repertoires in general were vast and sophisticated — giving the lie to the old nonsense about ignorant peasants who could hardly summon a note or count their toes. It is in the light of this historical background that the Hermetic musical model should be examined.

Before taking the examination further, we should also consider the simple fact that *we are no longer playing or hearing the same scales and modes as were our ancestors.* This is not the regular musicological discussion about the true order or intervals of the so-called 'Greek Modes', [5] but a much simpler matter altogether. During the last two centuries or so, the gradual tempering and adjustment of musical pitch ratios and intervals has changed the character of the music that we hear or play. It is no longer identical with the music that nature produces in the unadulterated human voice, or in the harmonic sequences shown by simple acoustic experiments.

Modern musicians who revive old works and old instruments enjoy the strident and expressive tone colour of replicas of period instruments, but they seldom take the trouble to play the actual intervals which would have been produced, unless these are an unavoidable property of the physics or acoustic of the design. This revival of early music is particularly prone to problems when vocal material is attempted, as the modern trained singer is conditioned to sing 'out of tune' relative to the natural intervals produced by the human vocal apparatus. Art is no longer the Ape of Nature.[6]

The acoustic evidence of certain mathematical ratios or intervals of pitch between high and low notes was regularly used by philosophers, alchemists, mystics and magicians, as well as in orthodox religious practice. The primary intervals or proportions of octave, fifth, fourth and third were assumed to be suggestive of a deeper universal proportion and

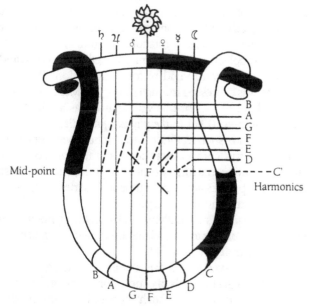

Fig. 5   The Lyre of Apollo

harmony.[7] From the pagan music of the lyre of Apollo[8] (see Fig. 5) to the refined speculations of Robert Fludd and Athanasius Kircher, to the modern and practical expositions of Steiner in connection with music and rhythm in human nature, Hermetic musicologists have not hesitated to merge the natural and the divine, inspiration and acoustics, physics and metaphysics. To such thinkers the natural musical intervals were clear evidence of higher order of relativity, corresponding to their mystical or religious leanings.

Modern physics, since the work of Albert Einstein and his successors, tends towards startlingly similar conclusions, though the initial premises may be very different indeed. It is interesting to observe in this context that the Hermetic writers of the sixteenth, seventeenth and eighteenth centuries were attempting to express a musical model which had been intentionally suppressed by the Church at an early date — although that same Church had inherited the model from classical Greek and Roman sources, plus the more clearly Eastern influences of Gnostic, Hebrew and various other sources now difficult to define. This suppression was not entirely aimed at a spiritual leavening of the laity's musical consciousness, but more concerned with an intentional control of the keys to magical or invocatory power in connection with actual acoustics — particularly those of the human voice.[9]

In the works of Kircher (a Jesuit), Fludd (an Anglican), Michael Myer and numerous other philosophers or alchemists both well known and obscure, acoustic properties, rotations of number series and mystical or religious symbolism are wilfully mixed together, correlated and utilized, often with powerful and vivid pictorial illustrations.[10]

The divine was expressed through music (the Muse), not as a personal or individual creativity (for this was regarded as a reflection of Grace or Divine Inspiration) *but in the physical properties of sound itself.* This is why great minds such as Fludd and Kircher spent time playing with numerical patterns, composition devices in the form of charts, tables, or actual computing machinery (one such by Kircher still exists), fugue patterns and progressions of numerical series, without actually 'composing' in the modern accepted sense.

It is facile to dismiss such dallying as obsessive or ignorant, particularly when the critic is unable to unravel the connections suggested in Hermetic literature and put them to work!

As we have observed earlier, this inability to activate the Hermetic or alchemical or magical models of conception or energy lies not with the stupidity of the originators of such models, but with the difficulty in relating such models to the modern modes of awareness and conscious activity. Many of the Hermetic researchers were the greatest thinkers and questioners of their era. Some, such as Newton or Kepler, inscribed their names and theories upon the foundation stones of modern astronomy and physics, not by a sudden flux of rational thought, but through work with astrology, mystical and metaphysical harmonic theories, number series, and other Hermetic conceptual models.[11] The resulting theories about the solar system have had a powerful and lasting effect right into the present century.

The models from which such discoveries were deduced were directly derived from pagan magical originals, the ritual practices of the Greeks and Romans, and the later mystical and mathematical systems of Qabalah that permeated Europe from the middle ages onwards. More obscure to the modern researcher, but no less important, is the potent inheritance of non-classical, non-oriental philosophy and belief, native to Europe, that of the peoples loosely known as 'the Celts'. Upon these models, the classical and Christian developments were grafted, and the roots still show clearly in folklore and traditional beliefs in the present day. Even modern 'Celtic' traditional music, from Scotland, Ireland, Brittany, Galicia and parts of Wales shows occasional conscious use of quarter-tone intervals and complex rhythms, undeniably ancient and primal elements of music which have been lost in the modern homogenized musical conception.[12]

To the Hermetic writers of the sixteenth to eighteenth centuries, music of the sort described was a commonplace occurrence; it was the music of the *majority*, if we accept musicological and cultural evidence, and not a decaying aspect of a disappearing cultural minority.

A careful consideration of the cultural context of folk musics and folklore in connection with alchemical, Hermetic and Rosicrucian publications will bear a great deal of fruit.

It soon becomes clear to the student of the musical theories suggested in Hermetic literature that either the faith of the authors was of the mountain-moving variety, or that important keys to the understanding and activation of the systems offered have been lost. This becomes more than painfully obvious when we consider the disreputable literature of ritual magic, most of which appears to be utter nonsense.

The world-view, the central themes and theories, all fall apart in the cold light of modern physics and acoustics, when the experimental evidence fails to live up to the psychological theories offered. The proportions of octave, fifth and third, for example, may indeed be representative of religious or mystical symbolism in the imagination of the writer, but they cannot be utilized in music to transfer such realms of altered consciousness objectively to all listeners. Nor, of course, is any experiment infinitely repeatable under identical conditions.

As a result of this apparent failure, it is assumed that we cannot understand the models offered by the Hermetic and mystical writers, merely because they themselves did not really understand the true implications of their own theories. Alternatively, they must have taken on faith many obvious inconsistencies in their theories, and never attempted to resolve them consciously.

Religion, however, was not the only key that released the visions of the ancients, or of the Hermetic philosophers.

The keys to the Hermetic musicology, and to many other aspects of magic and metaphysics which are not directly under discussion are found in the realization of apparently higher orders of shape or pattern, applied in practice through natural acoustics.

This principle of *application* is very important indeed, as by such action, the alchemist, magician or mathematical visionary attempted to save, purify or redeem the physical elements which were supposed to have devolved from certain metaphysical originals as taught by ancient tradition. Personality in composition of music through such systems was irrelevant, as there was already a special or spiritual power hidden therein, which could be brought out to rebirth by structuring the physical sounds in relationship to the metaphysical master-patterns or archetypes which occupied the consciousness of the human mediator.

Inspiration, in the form of a gift of altered states of awareness, could occur through the repetition of regular musical structures *used as acoustic symbols*. This was identical to the theories that applied to ritual, meditation, prayer and creative visualization in contemplation. Eccelesiastical plainchant is supposed to operate in exactly this manner, as is the music and chanting of many Eastern monastic and magical orders. This method is not merely one of hypnotic repetition, but stems from that same ancient musical 'system' that permeates world folk music, and which is intimately related to certain natural patterns of the human psyche and biochemistry.

What type of model, let us ask, can be applied to music in general, to activate it in the manner suggested by the Hermetic philosophers? The answer is this: a very simple step-by-step assembly of basic musical-numerical concepts, transferred through the ancient Elemental Circle into symbols of *shape*; the shapes are then expressed as *sound*.

Practice with this musical model will reveal some insights into other more complex systems or models, and into the general relationship between magic, metaphysics and music in early writings and actual use. This is not a definitive or master model, but is a simple and broad-range key which is easily understood without recourse to the support of complex mathematics. Indeed, in Hermetic use of music, the complex relationships are implicit, as they are in actual acoustics, and need not be applied for effective use, as they are devolutions of primary original relationships. Careful consideration of this model will also give considerable insight into some of the apparent problems in a sympathetic interpretation of alchemy, magical symbolism and the Qabalah.

Most important, however, is our present *musical* study, and the model offered will provide a rather refreshing way of considering music; a viewpoint which has been virtually lost in the welter of conflicting issues and interpretations of the art and its role in modern life. The model may be applied without 'religious' or 'mystical' convictions, and even the non-musician will be able to conduct simple vocal or keyboard experiments with the system illustrated. By attempting such experiments we are supporting the beliefs of the Hermetic philosophers, who claimed that the intellect was the servant of the higher orders of consciousness, and that use of intellect would bring out these higher functions regardless. The proviso must be, of course, that they applied intellect or logic to their pure visions, rather than to the pursuit of materialist or trivial ends.

As with all broad symbolic systems that affect awareness, results will vary according to the spirit in which the system is applied. To the intellectual or logical and mathematical person, many new and amusing ways of writing or formulating music may be discovered, in addition to an intriguing system for interpretation of existing music. For the creative artist, the system offers a new tool for shaping music according to inspiration. To the poet, mystic or religiously inclined individual, it offers many insights into the expression of the intuitions regarding the divine, and it is in this manner that the old writers intended their expositions to be applied. They were not prepared to divide the natural and the divine, but sought to clarify the unity between them, which had become clouded in human perception.

6.

The Model

Preparing the Hermetic Speculum or Magical Mirror of Music
We begin with the basis of the Four Elements, a conceptual model of
existence which has been applied from the most ancient of times up
to the present day, in both Eastern and Western cultures. Although a
great deal of literature has dealt with the Four Elements, we must briefly
reconsider them before we assemble the component parts of our Hermetic
Speculum or Musical Mirror.

The Elements, Air, Fire, Water and Earth, were idealized archetypes
of aspects of existence. Though they were supposed to manifest as their
obvious physical counterparts, they also permeated all existing matter
and consciousness and energy, regardless of the relatively impermanent
outer appearance or subjective quality. Curiously, this viewpoint is no
longer in conflict with materialist physics, but it is important not to confuse
the Elements with the chemical *table of elements*, which is a sub-system
derived from a restatement of alchemical experiments.[1]

In synthetic or synchronistic metaphysical systems, all modes or aspects
of being are related to certain basics: the Elements. These emerge from
whatever origin is postulated by religious belief or intuition, and have
parallels throughout human religious or metaphysical systems.

As we have explained above, a religious foundation is quite unnecessary
for application of our Hermetic model, and the Four Elements may be
understood as four principles of all observable phenomena, both objective
and subjective: Earth — *relative solidity*; Water — *relative fluidity*; Fire —
relative incandescence; and Air — *relative insubstantiality*. These four relative
states or rates apply to human awareness as effectively as they apply
to material existence. The nature of the Elements is such that they are
states of *relationship*, and not separate entities in isolation.

Fig. 6 shows a typical example of the pattern of relationship of the

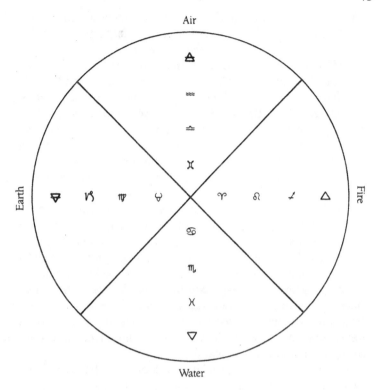

Fig. 6 The Four Elements

Four Elements, with various attributes of relationship. This diagram is merely one of many similar illustrations, ranging from extremely basic to extremely obscure and incomprehensible systems, which have shown the Four Elements through the ages in pictorial form.

Contrary to popular belief, the aim of alchemy or of magic was not that of compelling the natural world to serve the operator, but to alter the apparent confusion of the Elements in the outer or fallen world and so cause them to revert to a primary or divine mode of relationship. This was to be achieved through the utterance of words of power or by fabricating the Philosopher's Stone. The result would be the redemption of the natural world through the mediation of humankind.

In Hermetic musicology, the operator aimed to produce a musical pattern that attuned as closely as possible to the divine archetype. The theory was held that such a successful attunement would act through the physical (acoustic) vibrations that carried it, and cause actual changes in the consensual fabric of apparent reality.

Modern notions of 'pleasure', 'entertainment', 'creative genius' or 'emotional inspiration' were absent from such a musical model, and may even have been disdained by the practitioners. Monastic music of the present day still consists of repetitions of specific musical patterns, linked to liturgical texts. Although understanding of the system has been lost or suppressed, it is still applied within strict rules and limitations.

It is not too unreasonable to suggest that an application of the Hermetic music system given in the following pages will produce results in the modern listener, particularly if the listener is also the performer, and especially if the performance is given with the unaffected human voice.

After careful consideration of Fig. 6 we should include musical notes in the collection of attributions. Those who disagree with the collection offered may leave out whatever they do not like, providing they grasp the main sequence of fourfold relationship, or the Four elements.[2] In practice, systems of this type become most effective if the individual draws up lists of correspondences initially, and then begins to observe the Elements within themselves and within outer phenomena, but such application is not necessary for an understanding of the musical system during the initial stages of learning.

Further musical attributes with general parallels that extend beyond musicology, are important in the assembly of the Elemental sequence: Air *begins;* Fire *accelerates;* Water *culminates;* Earth *concludes.*

Before we approach the attribution of actual notes of music, the reader should be reminded that any such notes are arbitrary, and that the *relationship* or *shape* is the primary factor of importance. In other words, because our musical examples begin upon the note C or the note G, does not suggest for one moment that this actual pitch is inherent in the Element to which it is ascribed.

There are several theories of pitch related to Elemental or magical levels of existence, but no conclusive proof as to their accuracy. To grasp the matter fully, the question of 'pitch' should be ignored, and the effect of 'relationship' given full attention. Remember, we are not hearing or using natural intervals in our modern music, and our standard pitch has changed several times within the last century or so. The value of an alternative musicology lies not in absolute attributes, for such attributes actually cannot exist, but in a fresh approach to the relationships inherent in the natural scales or patterns of ascent and descent in music that is common to humankind.

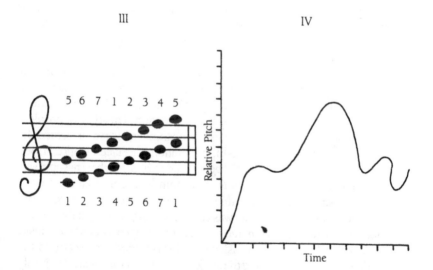

I   The Elements in 'Fifths'
II The Elements as Numbers
III The Musical Scale and its Fifth in numbers
IV Graph of Pitch and Time extension

Fig. 7 The Elements as Numbers, Pitch and Time

Our examples will be in tones and semitones, the standard intervals that have developed in Western music in recent times. But we could just as well use quarter tones, which are known in Western traditional music, natural vocal intervals, and are still used fully in Eastern music to the present day. Perhaps the simplest way of visualizing music is as a graphic display, pitch intervals relative to duration. This is the only true uni-directional or linear way of displaying a musical passage in visual terms, and has been adopted by musicologists in recent years, particularly in the expression of traditional music, which has many pitch, decoration and rhythmic aspects which cannot be represented by the severely limited standard notation system (see Fig. 7).

In the final analysis, when all educational preconceptions are removed, music is really a set of numbers, in varied modes or sequences. In Hermetic musicology, this has always been realized, and the numbers are arranged and rearranged in certain meaningful rotations, which are expressed as musical scales of arbitrary pitch designation.

For mere convenience, we shall use the basic 'major scale' common in Western music, the mode of seven notes ascending and descending between given octaves of a primary named note. This scale should be familiar to most people, either vocally or instrumentally, and is so ingrained in the Western consciousness that almost anyone can sing a 'major scale'.[3]

The modern alterations of temper or relativity between notes are mainly due to certain mechanistic problems in the development of keyboard instruments, and in the interesting difficulties that arise when various instruments of music are played in combination. This type of problem was of major importance to the Hermetic thinkers, as it represented the dissonance or lack of relationship inherent in the 'fallen world'. Robert Fludd,[4] for example, produced diagrammatic tables which were supposed to enable the user to apply or avoid certain harmonic relationships in playing or singing. By Fludd's time, however (early seventeenth century), the general direction of music was already drifting away from the ancient modal or sequential system into what later developed as 'classical' music.

Alchemical or mystical musicology of this period may seem, to the modern student considering the subject in retrospect, to attempt to justify itself in terms of harmonic or classical form, but the concepts are rooted in modal or rotational patterns, not in corrected or rationalized polyphony.

The reader should now work patiently through our examples, trying to set aside all musical intellectual conditioning and preconception, in an attempt to relate to an alternative musical model. Most of the concepts involved are childlike (but not childish) basic, and easily accessible. Indeed, they were so self-evident to the Hermetic writers, that they have often been ascribed as great 'secrets' that were hidden away, and much nonsense speculated about their nature. Many clues were scattered throughout texts in publication that lead to simple concepts, such as those applied to music in our present model.

The Four Elements as Musical Notes

We will use the scale of C major: C D E F G A B C. Earth is the 'heaviest' element, so it naturally relates to the lowest note of C. Water is next in relative substantiality, with the note D. Fire relates to E, and Air to F.

With these four steps up the ladder, we have covered one-half of the basic scale.

We could express the steps neutrally as numbers: 1, 2, 3, 4. A numerical

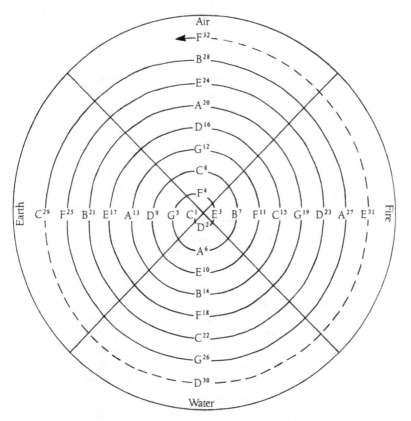

Fig. 8 The Expanding Spiral of Music

comparison avoids musical preconceptions about pitch, providing the rotation of the number sequences is retained: Earth, 1; Water, 2; Fire, 3; Air, 4. To complete the scale, we make a second revolution of the circle of relationships: Earth, G/5; Water, A/6; Fire, B/7; Air, C/8.

If we continued this process into a further octave, we would generate a spiral of relationships, as in Fig. 8.

Before *Earth* is expressed as the note C for a second time, the spiral is turned through four octaves, or numbers 1 to 28. Examination of this spiral will show a series of basic relationships as found in music, but in itself it is insufficient, as it only forms *one part* of the set of relationships that are implicit in a Hermetic musical model. The spiral can be turned indefinitely, returning to Earth/C at the beginning of every eighth revolution.[5] This sequence is the original pattern from which active Elemental energies or relationships are generated.

In the conceptual model which underpins the type of system employed by the Hermetic philosophers, alchemists and metaphysicians, all constituent parts are reduced to their simplest components, the numbers 1 to 4, or the Four Elements.

If we do this with the musical notes, we are left with CDEF in our chosen mode or scale. This sequence is one half of the octave, Earth, Water, Fire, Air. If we consider the four-fold sequence as a graphic shape, we discover that CDEF has the same contour as GABC. In music, they make harmonies with one another, giving the interval known as the perfect fifth (Fig. 7).

In Hermetic terms, the application of the notes CDEF is identical to the application of the notes GABC, as they are related to one another through relative shape, pitch and harmony. A study of basic acoustics will also show that they are inherent in one another as parts of the *harmonic sequence* which occurs whenever a note is produced. This inherent harmony was extremely significant, and was thought to be natural to all existence, as it could be proven in music.

For the reader who wishes to pursue the metaphysical implications of our musical theory, it should be stated that the system is an open one and not a closed cycle. It is this assumption that the Hermetic writers employed closed cycles in their symbolism that has led to confusion over many aspects of interpretation. The musical or mathematical models were used as means of communicating perceptions or states of awareness that were non-verbal and difficult to explain in written form. The illustrations, paradoxes, systems and number codes were created to generate a leap or jump of consciousness, to jolt the perception over specific barriers into areas previously unknown to the traveller. When the systems used degenerated into closed and utterly formulated sequences, they lost their value, and became mere shells. Astrology is an excellent example of such a system, wherein its widespread popularity is due to rule-of-thumb prediction; the more subtle aspects which are recognized by good astrologers are nevertheless based upon cycles of synchronicity which are not understood. Perhaps we should be fair, and state that both physics and chemistry may also be summarized in the same manner.

It might be assumed that to activate the Elements inherent in the musical scale or half scale, we should compose suitably evocative or invocatory music, but as has been suggested above, the Hermetic musicology looks for such music in number sequences which are said to represent higher orders of existence. Setting aside the discussion of the existence of such orders, which has been continuing for many thousands of years, we may still examine the system used to obtain the number sequences.

Traditionally, the seven notes of the scale are attributed to the seven planets known to the ancients. These created the well-known 'Music of the Spheres', a proportional symbology which was applied to geocentric and heliocentric concepts of the solar system, and which strongly influenced the development of modern astronomy.

It remains to demonstrate how the Elemental system and the planetary system are related. Various attempts have been made to achieve this unified theory, which ultimately rests upon a foundation of spherical geometry and structures such as the famous Platonic solids, rather than on literary juggling with tables of correspondence.

In basic magical or metaphysical models of Creation, a simple number sequence is used as an analogy of processes which are beyond normal conception or understanding. If we literally apply these analogous principles, in the most simplistic manner possible, we will be duplicating the development of the models used by the Hermetic writers and thinkers.

Squaring the Circle

To bring our musical mirror out into acoustic expression, we first need to *square the circle*. This ancient problem is featured in several ways in metaphysics, from very simple examples such as those that follow, to complex magical squares which have never been solved or translated, such as those of the cryptographer Dee who worked for Queen Elizabeth I of England. (Although claims have been made to translation of Dee's systems, they are not by any means accurate, complete or even intelligible).

Although we have referred the reader to some rather abstruse concepts, no knowledge of mathematics is necessary to follow the suggestions given

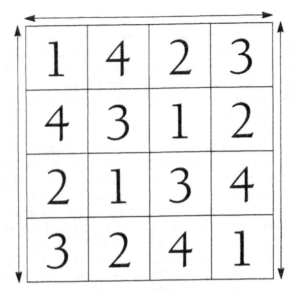

Fig. 9   Elemental Square as Numbers

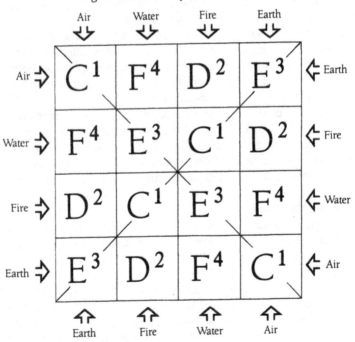

Fig. 10   Elemental Square as Music

in Fig. 9, which uses only the numbers 1 to 4.

In this case, we do not 'add up' the magical squares, but we play or sing them, giving one note of our scale to each number.

This gives us Fig. 10 and four Elemental musical sequences or calls.

Each sequence is the result of relating the basic four numbers in a changing order, whereby the initial order of 1234 or 4321 is regarded as a foundation from which the changes or rotations are generated. It can be seen immediately from the square that pairs of opposites occur between Air/Earth and Water/Fire.

Once again, we will remind the reader that this is not a definitive system, merely an example of how such systems are generated.

To apply these musical phrases, we assign them to the basic Elemental Circle, using one call or phrase to each quarter. The basic spiral of octaves shows immediately that seven notes are implicit or passive in each Elemental quarter. They are activated by specific combinations, such

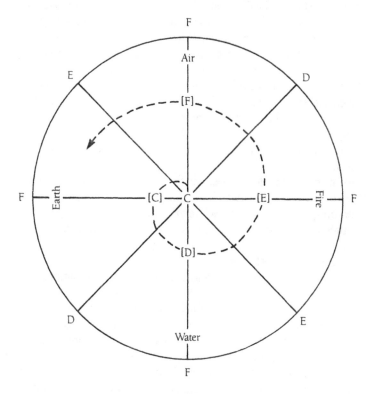

Fig. 11 Music in Potential

as those derived from the number-square used in our example.

If we follow our musical scale faithfully, we can allocate the root note C not only to each Element in turn as it spirals through the octaves, but also as a central drone or pedal note, upon which all the various possible harmonies are formed. This would be shown by Fig. 11.

In this illustration, we have another key diagram of potentials, an idealized state of balance between our Four Relative Units. One note remains at the centre, while the other three mark potential relationships which are unactivated or unconnected. This corresponds to the 'Undifferentiated' metaphysical state, represented in various ways by different schools of symbolism.

The Spiral of Fig. 8 represents the apparent steps of Creation within a two-dimensional analogy, exactly as we represent the steps of the musical scale from which our music is formed. This spiral, however, is only the result of our limited perception, and the Elemental patterns, the Four Relative Divisions of the Circle, are actually a flat representation of a Sphere, composed of Three Rings or Circles. In other words, according to the Hermetic conception, we *think* that music is made up of graded steps or scales, but these are actually an illusion of continuity derived from other patterns which we cannot usually perceive.

The value of all our number games, magical squares, superimposition of diagrams, etc., is not a literal attempt to juggle various factors and force them to fit with religious preconceptions. It is an analogous attempt to indicate how Creation might occur from a combination of Active and Passive Principles; and then it is reduced to deliberate absurdity in application of musical sequences.

If the reader wishes to discover whether or not these sequences actually *do* alter human consciousness, he or she should experiment with singing or chanting each Call in turn, while visualizing or meditating upon the attributes and qualities of the Element which it represents.

Retrieving the Planets

Finally, we retrieve the Seven Planets in the following manner.

1. Attribute a note or defined pitch for each Element, commencing at the lowest note of the chosen group for the Element of Earth. This escalating spiral pattern is music as perceived from the serial or human world of time values. It is linear, and produces basic harmonic relationships as it spirals upwards or downwards: Fig. 8.
2. Using a number sequence which indicates possible interrelationships between the basic notes, we create a table or key which offers four

representative calls or shapes which may be expressed as musical phrases.

Each of these calls represents one Element, and the correlation between the patterns of notes also shows the polarity of opposites within the Elements themselves: Figs. 9 and 10.

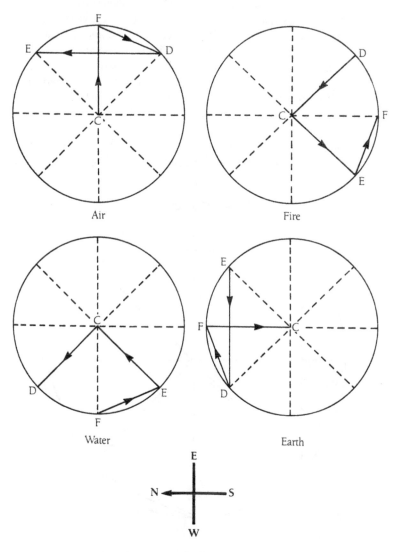

Fig. 12 Musical glyphs of the Elements

3. Apply the key, which is merely a way of expressing certain number combinations inherent in the numbers 1-4 (i.e. seemingly part of the fabric of existence as we perceive it) to the potential field, which acts as the blank surface for our Hermetic Speculum. This is Fig. 11 which is an analogy of potential states of existence which have not been polarized or energized; undifferentiated music.
4. The resulting *glyphs* or *sigils* are shown in Figs. 12-14. These diagrams show us a symbolic pattern for each Element, and indicate how these Elements combine within an(unlimited) spherical field to create *The Tree of Life*. The Tree of Life includes the Seven Planets within its system, and our Hermetic musical key links the Elements and the Planets in an actual and acoustic system, which may be used for chanting, composition or musical analysis.

The present explanation of this system, and the principles from which it is derived, is necessarily short. There are many conclusions to be drawn

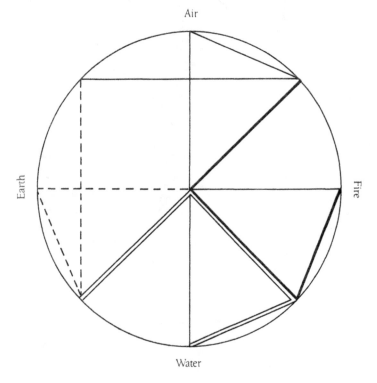

Fig. 13 First Combination of the Elements

by further ramifications of number, geometry, harmonics and traditional magical and Hermetic and Qabalistic symbolism which will occupy the mind of the curious reader. Most of these ancient and little-understood systems are not directly explicable by regular intellectual or logical effort, but are derived from keys such as the above, which may help to explain many of the indecipherable codes, keys and symbolic sequences used in manuscript, in print and in traditional exposition.

Most important of all, they represent a means of applying the metaphysical concepts as units *which may be directly communicated*. There is no form of communication as pure and as generally open to transmission as music, and if any of the old writer's theories about the

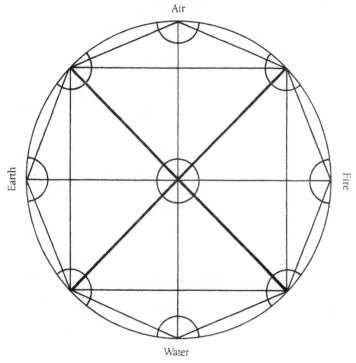

The musical elements in the full octave

(1) The Circle is Squared
(2) The Elements are unified
(3) A Perfect Tree of Life is generated
(4) The Planets relate harmoniously

Fig. 14 A Full Cycle of Musical Elements

nature of reality are correct, we may find them most practically applied in the musical clues which have been handed down to us from time immemorial.

These clues were finally set out in written form at a time when it was clear that the traditional corpus of teaching regarding reality (which encompasses religion, magic, physics, chemistry, metaphysics, philosophy, music, poetry, art, dance and theatre) was about to be fragmented by the generation of a new wave of consciousness, that of the 'Age of Reason'. In the twentieth century, we live among the problems and benefits which manifested from that wave of Reason and Experiment, and the Spiral (symbolized by the spiral of octaves) is turning towards a re-evaluation of metaphysical and even magical theories, as they begin to be supported by the remarkable discoveries of modern physics, biology and psychology.

If you have conducted the experiment successfully, and made an inner realization of the Musical Mirror, it will come alive for you within your own imagination, and may lead to realizations and affinities with other branches of the metaphysical or esoteric arts and sciences. On the other hand, you may wish to restrain your application to the therapeutic or creative aspects of music, and in this area alone the model will repay continual use.

Traditionally, alchemical experiments were repeated many times, and this repetition reflects the organic nature of the Hermetic sciences. Far from attempting to prove that an experiment could be repeated infinitely with identical results (something which is no longer claimed, even by materialist sciences other than for rule-of-thumb tolerances in application) the Hermetic metaphysicians knew that an experiment changed fractionally with every operation. How could it be otherwise? The seasons move, the stars change, the sun and the earth alter their relative positions with every beat of our artificial measurement of time . . . nothing can ever be repeated under identical circumstances, only under harmonically related circumstances. We find this in physical music, where the spiral of intervals expands slightly with every new turning, although we contract to fit with our human requirements expressed through the various systems of temperament.

Repetition of a magical, psychological or metaphysical exercise is not merely reiteration. It moulds and regenerates consciousness under a spiralling set of inner and outer relationships that change constantly. Musicians know this through the discipline of their physical practice; eventually the hands take care of themselves and new creative realizations come to life through the music that the hands are playing. Yet such a deep interaction between human and music could not have been possible without hours of repetition, each repeated event being slightly different from the previous one.

The very basic musical patterns used to build up the Mirror, or the Tree of Life, are not mere steps to be left behind. This simplicity is the simplicity of foundational units that may be built into very profound and complex structures, and the structures are harmonic entities found in human consciousness and in the Macrocosmic consciousness which esoteric and religious traditions assert to be a higher octave of our own.

Once the Mirror is assembled, it may revitalized within your own imagination, and eventually carry awareness into the realms hinted at by the ancient writers, by mystics, and by the implications of developing science.

7.

Chanting and the Power Centres

This chapter will seem highly speculative to some readers; while the musical motifs or Elemental Calls have a psycho-biological relationship to a number of modern researches, the theory of the power centres or tone centres is entirely traditional, and begins where science or medicine cease to speculate. It has some close analogies with the practice of acupuncture, which defines a set of energetic pathways or meridians within the human life-structure, yet carries even this definition further, for it specifies that the energies are directly affected by will, by controlled operation of consciousness itself.[1]

Such traditions are said to be very ancient indeed, and the oriental parallels are known to be thousands of years old. In the West, we have less concrete evidence of established systems, but a scattering of lore remains, filtered through classical sources or through oral tradition. The theory of the power centres or tone centres is found stated quite clearly in a number of alchemical or theosophical Renaissance illustrations, which represent a formal restatement of an oral or almost underground tradition. We may presume, without any firm evidence, that a science of this sort is preserved within the Catholic Church, and not entirely through the specialized developments of the Jesuit order, but from earlier monastic traditions. Such traditions in turn echo the remnants of pagan teachings on the energetic link between the human body and the human psyche.[2]

Medieval sources, such as the *Prophecies of Merlin* (twelfth century) seem to preserve oral poetical traditions in which the inner powers are demonstrated. They may represent the remnants of a Druidic or native Celtic wisdom teaching, presented in a garbled but still accessible form.[3]

Whatever the historical or cultural origins of such systems, no one can deny their persistence . . . if they are utterly spurious they reappear in each century with surprising regularity; they are an inherent set of intimations, something which floats up from the depths of the consciousness into varied theoretical expressions. As such there can be little doubt that the theory of the power or tone centres has some intuitive grounding in the interplay between awareness and the flow of energy through the physical body.[4]

In the metaphysical and magical traditions which preceded modern psychology, the *imagination* was of paramount importance. It is the controlled imagination (moulding of consciousness into sets of images by an act of will) that acts as the fertile medium in which the obscure theories spring to life as real experiences.

This most emphatically does not mean that it is all an idle fantasy, for the image-making ability of humans is their most potent power; your image of yourself (as modern psychology repeatedly asserts) has remarkable effects upon your mind and body. In traditional or magical psychology the imagination is employed as the ground (Earth) which is moulded by will and practice into matrices for inherent life energies.

The physical body is often said to be the element of Earth, man moulded of red clay,[5] but it is esoterically the expression of all four Elements shaped through the imagination. As we image, so we express. The imagination is one of the highest harmonics of the Element of Earth, in the old elemental psychological/magical systems.

So when the argument 'Ah, but it is all imaginary' is heard, it does not invalidate the theory in any way. A trained or disciplined imagination is very different from an idle or dissipated one; exercises of the sort described form the basic training for the development of the imagination as a powerful tool. Ultimately the imagination creates the outer world, by moulding the energies that go to build up that world through specific matrices. Our first experience of this power is, of course, within ourselves.

The method of operation shown in the diagrams and text is slightly different from that usually published, as it represents an 'inner' or 'secret' system, though all such secrets are quite open to a properly attuned image-making consciousness. It is a harmonic system, as is proper for a study of esoteric consciousness and music, and not a religious or dogmatic or cult practice. We may be Christian or pagan, and still employ our imaginations in work of this sort without offending God or the Goddess. In this context it should be remembered that the alchemical or Hermetic writings were often produced by fervent Christians, and that the esoteric Grail lore remained within a highly orthodox medieval culture, yet both preserved conscious and unconscious levels of magical technique.

But even the materialist or atheist may experiment with the imagination. Indeed, such a person has distinct advantages in some respects, for he or she may be able to approach the exercises with a consciousness free of religious conditioning. Furthermore, if you have even a fragment of active imagination,[6] this type of discipline will always work, given the hard fact of effort on your part. Ultimately the interaction between human energies and vocal tones moulded by the imagination is natural — it is of nature. We can therefore cast all concepts of magic, pagan, Christian and so forth out of the window and merely work with the system suggested.

How to Use the Theory
The material is in a concentrated and direct form, and a few notes on its general use will be helpful.

1. Read through the entire system or pattern several times, until you are familiar with its development.
2. Try the exercises in a quiet room where you will not be disturbed; this simple basic essential is, in itself, almost a guarantee of eventual success. The imagination and the subtle energies require an uninterrupted space and time in which to come fully alive.
3. Avoid the use of television while working with these exercises; by externalizing the image-making faculty (television) the flow of the energies which are employed in the power centres is weakened.
4. Follow the musical advice given in our appendix on 'Listening to Music'.
5. When you are familiar with the material, work on the awakening of the first three centres or vocal tones (Earth, Water, Fire). The student can only progress to the higher centres when the three primary centres have some degree of flexibility and development. There is nothing coy or secretive or 'occult' about this limitation; we would not try to lift heavy weights or run a marathon race without some preliminary training and warm-up; the human body does not suddenly mature into adult form, it *grows towards it*. Both of these analogies apply to the use of the power centres and vocal tones. A gentle harmonic progression will work; a rushed imbalanced attempt will not.
6. Try to keep a brief diary of your physical subjective and imaginative reactions to the exercises. This will help you to define your own development, and to become systematic in your visualizations.
7. To gain even the most modest result, a short regular period of work

is needed daily. Fifteen to twenty minutes is sufficient, but five is not.

8. Do not attempt these exercises while taking any sort of drug or medication (including tobacco, alcohol, marijuana). They simply do not work with chemical filters in operation, and we can easily fool ourselves while imbalanced by drugs within the bloodstream.

9. Do not attempt to practise popular oriental methods of meditation adapted for European-American use while working these special exercises. No musician would expect to play the piano and the harp at the same time, or the sitar and the violin. They are all musical instruments, they all use similar techniques, but skill develops with limitation and concentration upon one specific instrument at a time. In our example, the instrument is the specific model or system of power centres and vocal tones, derived from enduring esoteric Western traditions. It is a fine and responsive instrument, designed through long experience by many experts for our use. It also relates directly to our psychology and physiology, and our psychic inheritance from past cultures.

Visualization

In recent publications the use of visualization has been given an increasing emphasis; at one time this technique was a so-called 'occult secret', during the centuries of Christian suppression, while to early cultures life itself was enfolded and unified within a constant weaving of visions. We are now slowly returning to a restatement of that visionary faculty, at least as far as its value for psychic and physical well being. Magical or creative visualization carries the concept much further, but tends to be generalized and falsely unified in modern books, either psychological or metaphysical. There are a number of quite different faculties and styles and methods of creative vision, which need to be clarified for the student.

There is an unfortunate tendency for modern books to deal almost exclusively with dreamlike images . . . peaceful landscapes, inner adventures, floating journeys and so forth. While these are undoubtedly therapeutic in a mild sense, and a good introduction to levels of consciousness which are nowadays usurped by television and in danger of atrophy, we are not employing such visual images in our use of vocal tones and the power centres.

Visual images and the vocal tones

Many students experience a flush of images or mild fleeting glimpses of inner landscapes, people, symbols and other material during the early stages of these exercises; some do not see such images upon their inner field of vision, but in either case the dreamlike random images are not part of the technique. They belong to another related technique of composition or creative visualization, which is dealt with in a number of other books. The arising images should be regarded as a side-effect. They are neither important nor trivial; they merely occur during certain phases of development. There are a number of meditational centralizing or calming techniques which might be useful if the imagery persists to the exclusion of the proper work in hand, but a simple and continual reforming of the imagination within the basic symbolism described in the exercises is usually very effective.

As with all specialist methods, a certain amount of practice makes the working develop rapidly, and eventually the vocal tones themselves will attune the consciousness to their symbolic energies.

Do not be distracted by inner landscapes, and particularly do not waste your valuable exercise time and opportunity in idle drifting; this can be indulged in at other times of the day or through reading, and listening to imaginatively effective music. Television is not advised even as a recreation while working on these exercises.

In the traditional Elemental system, we are employing the imagination as an Earth power or energy (not to be confused with that of the planet Earth), and the vocal tones are therefore associated with the sense of touch just as much as with the sense of hearing. Both senses are really aspects of one sense and respond to different rates of vibration; the hearing responds to the acoustic vibrations of air, transmitted to the physical framework or its sensitive organs; the power centres begin to respond to the feeling or inner touch of the higher energies associated with the musical tone. In our musical analogy, we might define the physical musical note as C, D, E or F, while the inner energies are a higher octave or harmonic of that note, rotating through the Elemental spiral as shown in Fig. 8.

This analogy may help to define the generation of 'visions' during such inner exercises, for they belong to another cycle of tones upon a different level of the spiral. The first awakening of the power centres is *felt* (Earth, touching) rather than *seen* (Fire, light, seeing). The differences are only differences of rate of vibration, exactly as the differences between musical notes are only differences of rate of vibration. The musical analogy is extremely useful in inner arts or sciences, for it has a perfectly accessible outer expression as audible sound, mathematical formulae, and in many cases tangible vibration to the body. There are also many intangible musical vibrations which are sensed by our organisms but which do not necessarily become apparent to the regular outward-looking consciousness.

Eventually the perceptions are discovered to be effective variations of one unified perception; although we are able to state this intellectually, and even to define it scientifically, we are not usually able to realize this unity within our own consciousness. The general trend of progressive research or publication upon consciousness has been towards that fully defined but elusive unity; it may be religious, mystical, psychological or mathematical.

In the actual operation of metaphysics, we approach the unity through intentional operations of diversity, and the spiralling elemental model of music and consciousness should demonstrate this method and help us to widen the areas of our consciousness perception.

Taking a break

If the exercises become tiring or negative in any way, do not attempt to force them. One of the most interesting features of all creative work (be it music, art, poetry, scientific research, or metaphysics) is that a short pause at the right time will utterly transform the end result, bringing success where strenuous effort would have brought failure.

This is clearly indicated in the structure of the power centres themselves, for there is a transition point between the heart centre (Fire) and the throat centre (Air) at which a pause is often essential before further development can occur. Upon the Tree of Life, this pause is shown by the *Abyss*, a natural pulse or pause that is found between the realms of expressed consciousness and higher consciousness, or between the solar system and the greater universe, where the pause is that of the awareness encountering infinity. The bridge over this gap is a specific balanced mode of consciousness, and cannot be made by force, ignorance, false stimuli, or fear (Figs. 3 and 16).[7]

A break from the exercises will often enable the student to return with success, where previously the transition had been blocked. The pause, however, should not become an excuse for erratic practice; as in physical music, metaphysical vocal tones need regular rehearsal to mature fully.

None of the above rules are particularly hard to follow, and a willing attempt to work with the material along the lines described for a trial period will definitely produce results. To move beyond the first level of results takes a persistent and committed discipline, and a full use of the power centres and vocal tones may take years to enliven. As the method is organic or holistic, the results cannot be measured in limited terms. As the theory is a metaphysical one, the possibilities cannot be defined in mere words, but must be intuitively apprehended upon the Tree of Life itself.

As all of our musical-alchemical material has shown, we are the Tree of Life in the outer world, the inner world, and ultimately in the greater world of the macrocosm. But that pause is part of a different story — one which does not belong in this musical experiment.

Musical Notes and the Power Centres

A number of traditions regarding the power centres or 'psychic' centres of the body are very well publicized, usually deriving from Eastern authorities and methods. As music acts both physically and metaphysically to trigger or vibrate these centres on several levels, we should consider some basic simple attributes and theory for practical work.

As we are reinstating a Western esoteric system, one of great endurance and power, it is worth defining the vocabulary that will be used. The following is not the only system possible, nor is it offered as *the* true or genuine system; it is an established system, it works very effectively with a little regular discipline and practice, and it attunes to long-standing traditions of Hermetic, magical and metaphysical symbolism in the West.

The power centres
We shall be awakening five power centres; one for each Element, making four, plus the final confluence and radiance within the head of the meditator, which is often equated with the awakening Spirit. In our tradition they are not called psychic centres, as this term is often confused with spiritualism or mediumship, and it clearly does not employ the word 'psyche' either in the established classical sense, or in the modern altered terminology of psychology.

The centres are nodes of power, of life energy, that usually lie semi-dormant. They are intimately connected with our health and vitality, sexual attraction and orientation, and in some circumstances with the inner vision or power of seership. It is this last connection that has caused them to be called 'psychic' centres, but the inner vision is not necessarily the same as popular clairvoyance.[8]

If these centres are aroused and interconnected, they enable a through-flow of life energy in a highly amplified manner, which is traditionally employed to energize the inner faculties (mind and soul) to unfold into higher orders of consciousness. While in these higher states, a corresponding spiritual power is realized, which matches and harmonizes with the life energy of the power centres. The entire operation is known in the Western traditions as the *Arousal of the Inner Fire*, and is one of the central and essential practices of magic, mysticism, religious contemplation and practical metaphysics in all schools of inner or spiritual development.

A great deal of nonsense has been talked and written about this quite natural but rare organization of life-energies; it is not a great secret (least of all for sale), it is not a debased perversion (any more than any sexual or polar power may be pure or impure according to your own degree of grace or innocence) and it is not essentially dangerous, harmful or in any way imbalanced. As with any special training or energetic activity, from athletics through to dieting, a foolish, frivolous or obsessive use or development can generate problems, but these are the problems of the individual who abuses his or her energies, and not of the energies themselves.

The Four Centres have a general correspondence to physical locations in the body, and are often said to link to physical glands or nerve plexus areas. As there is a great deal of literature on this type of connection, we shall bypass it entirely, and define a very basic set of attributes, leaving the reader to make his or her own experiments and judgement of other connections that may or may not be present. Our system is based upon: the Four Elements; the Middle Pillar of the Tree of Life; and the Four Worlds (Figs. 15-16).

If we begin at the lowest physical location, this corresponds to the feet, which link to the element of Earth. The next is the generative organs, attuned to the element of Water. The third power centre equates to the heart, and the element of Fire. The fourth to the throat, and the element of Air. The fifth and last centre is in the forehead, and equates to the power of the living spirit, the summation of all the Four Elements and powers merged together.

Forehead *Spirit* (new cycle of illuminated consciousness)
Throat *Air* (utterance of the primal creative sound)
Heart *Fire* (human correspondence to solar energy)
Genitals *Water* (human correspondence to lunar energy)
Feet *Earth* (fundamental starting power and ground of being)

A number of further valuable attributes may be added to help our understanding of these power centres. We could, for example, visualize earth power rising up through our feet, meeting with our own generative power, and further rising to the heart, where it flames like the Sun, purifying our bloodstream. The energy then rises into the throat and attunes to our breath flowing in and out; finally it rises into the forehead, where it blossoms as an inner light and radiant force that radically alters our established modes of perception.

96

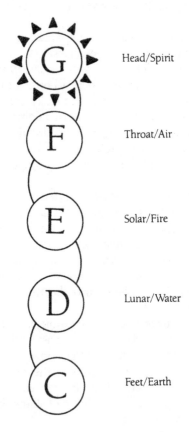

Head/Spirit

Throat/Air

Solar/Fire

Lunar/Water

Feet/Earth

Fig. 15 Music and the Power Centres

In musical symbolism, one note links to each power centre: Earth/C:
Water/D: Fire/E: Air/F: Spirit/G.

Basic use of the musical notes
The most easily developed method is to sit on a straight-backed chair,
with eyes closed, feet and hands uncrossed, in an upright but relaxed
position. Crossed legs or semi-lotus postures block the flow for this
exercise and cut off the basic Earth contact.

C/Earth: First we hum the basic note. This is called C for the sake of
argument, but you actually find your own C or ground drone note. It

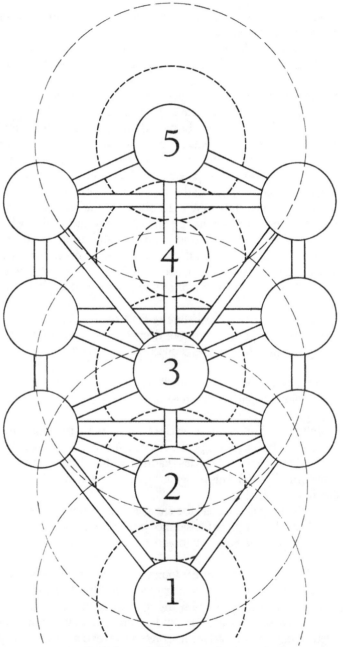

Fig. 16 Tonal Centres on the Tree of Life

is the lowest note that you can naturally reach, the one that feels right after a little experimentation.

While humming this note, we feel it vibrating and corresponding to a basic Earth power that flows through the feet and legs below the knees (Fig. 15).

To establish this power, the student must carefully meditate upon the symbols and concepts that relate to the element of Earth. This is a first stage of the work, and it cannot be passed over if success is truly sought.

The second stage is to meditate upon the Earth as a whole cycle of elements, the world of nature and of your own physical body, attuned to the generally disregarded powers that flow within physical matter, which live within the heart of the land and planet. This second stage corresponds to the Tenth Sphere (Kingdom) of the Tree of Life. In the first stage, we hummed the basic note (C) that resonates through our individual ground or Earth, and connected that to all Earth of the Elemental type or category. In the second stage we open this concept out into a cycle of all Four Elements, but each in the Kingdom or expressive world, making a complete entity or power pattern (Fig. 16).

Earth of Earth/Water of Earth/Fire of Earth/Air of Earth.
We utter the ground note (C or our deepest personal note) and feel it vibrating through the energies aroused by the meditation.

D/Water: The second power centre is *one whole tone* above the first (Fig. 15). This raises the pitch of our musical humming or chant; it modulates the energy into a new cycle.

As with the lowest centre and cycle of concepts, we progress through two stages: 1. The pure concept of Elemental Water. 2. The cycle of Water through all four elemental modes (Earth of Water/Water of Water/Fire of Water/Air of Water). This brings us to the lunar sphere or Foundation of the Tree of Life (Fig. 16).

As we change pitch, we feel the energies rising up into the region of the abdomen. They must be transformed by contemplation of the qualities and attributes of the Foundation and the Element of Water.

E/Fire: The third power centre is found by raising the pitch *by a further tone.* This corresponds to the element of Fire, the Sun, the Heart. As with the previous two centres, we raise the energies up the centre-line of the body through our visualization, and commence transforming them through a primary elemental meditation (on Fire) and a subsequent cycle of elements to make an entire unit. This corresponds to Beauty, the sixth sphere of the Tree of Life.

The power has now risen from Earth, to Water, to Fire, and practice with this system will generate a very real sensation of energy arising and transforming within the body. In general training, students are usually asked to concentrate on this threefold sequence (Earth, Water, Fire) before progressing further. There is no point in attempting to raise the pitch of our magical music or elevate the power centres higher, if the energy is not present in the first place. If the student feels that the power is arising and attuning as described, then he or she can progress to the last two phases, those of the throat and the head. If not, then repeated practice is necessary before working through the last two levels.

The transition

Our next stage, raising the power to the centre of the throat, is one of the most important magical and spiritual exercises in the metaphysical traditions. Up to this stage, we have been involved in the difficult task of arousing and attuning the earth, lunar and solar power centres, linking them together until they culminate in the Fire of the Heart.

So far, our meditational chant has been an echo, a faint reflection of the inner spiritual voice. If we have aroused the inner Fire correctly, we now give it a true voice, by bringing it into the throat. The power centre of the throat corresponds to the Abyss and the Bridge on the Tree of Life; it connects the Known and the Unknown by a slender thread. In our physical body this might correspond to the vocal chords, but esoterically it is found as a power centre that vibrates and makes its presence felt in the throat.

Some students feel a tightening of the throat, and a fear of choking when this first occurs, and many of the basic breathing exercises used in meditational training are designed not only for the general health of the individual but to prepare us for the awakening of the throat centre and the living Breath.

F/Air: Our fourth transition, therefore, is *one semitone*, a small step of quite distinctive character, an interval or change that has far-reaching consequences through all our music, both physical and metaphysical.

Firstly we raise the pitch of our chant, and meditate upon the element of Air as it moves in and out of the throat.

Secondly this is rotated through the cycle:

Earth of Air/Water of Air/Fire of Air/Air of Air.

During this phase, a distinct change in the vocal tone is often heard. The voice comes alive with a vibrant quality that has a powerful effect not only upon the meditator but upon listeners. Our individual voice has been enlivened by the arousal of the throat centre, which is our microcosmic image of the Voice of the Source of all Being. This change of tone quality can only happen from *within*. No amount of physical effort or training can gain it, and it is a magical event that derives from a spiritual power. It may occur very rapidly, or it may take many years; in either case the chanting and centring exercises may still be pursued and clarified.

The activation of the throat centre renders the effect of magical chanting more distinct and immediate. Once the throat comes alive, chants for the other centres become transferable to the listener, and also act with great speed for the meditator.

G/Spirit: The last power centre is that of the head, usually said to be located in the centre of the forehead. In many systems, particularly those of the East, a further centre is suggested, placed at the back of or above the head. This is shown in early Christian imagery as the halo of light around a holy man or woman's head.

For practical purposes, we shall concentrate on the centre of the forehead, as a successful opening of this power centre attunes to the spiritual locus represented by the halo.

In our ascending scale, the forehead is represented by the note G. This symbolizes a new cycle of spiritual music, as it is the first step of a new aspect of the rising notes of the chant. As we have seen in Chapter 6, the notes CDEF form an Elemental group (Air, Fire, Water, Earth), while G is the beginning of a new cycle. It is therefore both a higher form of Earth, and a new step into transformed consciousness.

In the standard Tree of Life, this connection is shown by the ancient teaching that the Crown, or top of the Tree, is identical to the Kingdom (Tenth or lowermost Sphere), but after a different fashion.

To raise our magical chant, based upon uttering the simple Five Tones, we visualize the energies converging and flowering in the forehead. Reactions to this exercise vary from a headache to an experience of intense illumination; and this illumination is the sign that the Inner Fire has been attuned by our magical chant.

The illuminated consciousness
The illuminated consciousness is not static; it is not a jolt or pleasure trip. In our context of magical chant, we are merely restating a body of age-old traditional wisdom teachings in simple modern language. The use to which this activated consciousness is put can vary according to the tradition employed. It may be part of worship, as in devotional chant,

or it may be directed by the structure of a prayer or magical ritual. We are summarizing in one brief section a subject that requires a complete book, and which can only be truly taught by direct tuition.

There is, however, one clear rule that will complete our exercise; the chant must be lowered, or relocated.

The most obvious manner of lowering the power focus is to chant back down the steps of the magical scale (G, F, E, D, C) finally bringing the consciousness back to its normal status, but this is always filled with surprises. When we draw the power back down, in this case by chanting, it passes through the power centres, carrying with it a resonance of spiritual energy, drawn from the higher worlds. This energy transforms or vitalizes each of the centres during its descent, and leaves one feeling more alive, fit and aware. In other words, *it changes the outer world,* in the form of our body/psychic complex.

This action works primarily within ourselves, but it can also take effect upon people, places, objects and other life forms. It is the *descending* chant or scale that carries the inner power outwards, while the *ascending* scale carries the outer consciousness inwards.

Magical or meditative chant, therefore, moves energy back and forward between modes of consciousness or Worlds, and there are points of transformation, acting like way-stations upon the route.[9] The main points are the ground note or tone (C) and the note one fifth above it (G); these correspond to the feet and the head in the human body, and to the Crown and the Kingdom upon the universal Tree of Life. The Crown represents origination, while the Kingdom represents expression; we cannot walk without the brain, nor can the brain move without the feet. The biological situation is the microcosmic reflection of a universal state; spirit is inherent and fulfilled within matter.

This is the most profound teaching of the Western Mysteries, and is, ultimately, the only spiritual teaching that endures all transitions, changes and states of relevant truth. In the ancient Mysteries it was stated as "Man, know thyself", while in modern physics it appears as the interchange of matter and energy at atomic or sub-atomic levels.

The mediating factor between spirit and matter is humankind, and we are able, by our utterances, to reflect the energies or Words that run through all existence, through all Worlds.

Our magical or spiritual application of shaped sounds and selected tones (music) is an expression of inner realities; such expressions may attune to the great figures of spiritual power such as Christ and Buddha, or may relate to the basic concepts of the Four Elements. With insight and practice, we can achieve a state of consciousness in which all varied symbols, powers, beings and energies, coalesce and resonate in harmony upon subsequent re-division.

Music shows this potential very clearly, in the simple fact that individual notes or tones may merge together as complex sets of relationships (chords) which in turn generate new patterns for the basic development of further creative shapes.

In classical European music this is achieved by the use of harmonies or chords that bring varied emphasis or meaning to melodic phrases, while in oral and Eastern traditions the same effect is gained by the methods of approach, delivery or departure from selected key notes or groups of notes. This second technique, which is well established in Western ethnic music, both black and white, is less rigid than the classical harmonic approach, and a merging of the two techniques represents one possible music of the future, in which the musical sound is represented in a non-linear manner. The circular or spherical maps used in metaphysics such as those briefly covered in our examples and exercises form a workable basis for a synchronous musical notation system.

8.

A Word of Power

One of the most misunderstood aspects of metaphysics and magic is the 'word of power'. As it is found in all religious, meta-psychological and transformational systems relating to consciousness, it is well worth including an example of one such 'word'. The use of traditional words of power is often found in the alchemical and Hermetic works generally associated with orthodox Christian or Hebrew religion; it is a worldwide intuitive and highly developed theory, and is not unique to any one religion, cult or geographical area. The word of power is a property of human consciousness, and is very closely attuned to the use of music, harmonic tones to alter consciousness, and the overall conception of an original creative Word or spiritual and unknown origin for all existence.

Most words of power were not spoken, but uttered at length — which means that they were musical. This extension of the vocal tone is equivalent to the extension of energy in the creation of the universe, but expressed through the limited form of human consciousness in the human world. Although the subject is shrouded in trivial mystery and easily derided as superstition, we have all heard and experienced words of power.[1]

Who can deny the power of a great orchestral chord? Who can deny the power of the opening sound of a highly amplified rock band? Who can deny the power of accelerating engine sounds? Yet these are all single acoustic 'words', complex vibratory patterns which result from input or powerful triggering impulses upon the medium of physical substances as the result of will. Another category of 'words' is found in the energetic sounds of the environment; the crash of a wave, the blast of wind; the rumble of falling rock. These represent not individual words of power, but harmonics of the Word of the World, or of the Four Elements, expressed in the outer Kingdom.

Traditional esoteric teaching holds that we all utter a reflection of the great Word continually, for we breathe in and out to remain alive. This inhalation and exhalation is said to be our harmonic of the great Breath, the originative power of which expands and contracts according to cycles beyond our limited comprehension. In modern physics we are beginning to formulate theories about such cycles, yet they were apprehended by intuition or metaphysical cognition thousands of years ago, and recorded in the sacred writings of both East and West. [2]

The reader who wishes to work only with the musical cycles and patterns of the main experiment need not be concerned with the theory of the word of power, but for those who wish to examine or perhaps attempt this advanced stage of musical metaphysics, the Word in our example is simple and represents a primal resonance inherent in human consciousness.

We know from the early Fathers of the Church that the common people of their time (the pagan peasants whom they sought to make into Christians) uttered ululations or jubilations, which were extended vowel sounds in a musical pattern. Such vocal utterances are still part of folksong today, though in the West they tend to be abbreviated or understated. These vocal sounds, free, expressive and highly communicative, are basic words of power. In the liturgy, they were developed and disciplined while being merged with approved texts; the result was plainchant. Such practices, however, did not appear in a vacuum, and were undoubtedly drawn not only from the musical chants of the people, but from the ritual use of the great pagan philosophies.

Any word has specific meaning; it is not merely a shaped utterance that arises on impulse. It may be repeated with many different levels of use and meaning all harmonic to its central concept; words of power are highly concentrated examples of this process.

Further Developments of the Vocal Tones and Words of Power
The reader will soon realize that the vocal tones, power centres, elemental calls and words of power are all interrelated, although they have been separated for technical and explanatory simplicity in our text. As has been said repeatedly in our earlier chapters, the entire process must be learned and developed in very simple easy stages; it cannot be merely assimilated intellectually and then put into practice.

We find the same problem in art music, where people are able to talk superficially about the subject without actually playing a note of music. For the musician it may take many years for the *wholeness* of music to shine through his or her particular instrument or technique.

In musical metaphysics, it is better to operate the basic experiments effectively than to attempt the more complex inner music or tones and words ineffectively.

There are some specific methods of combining vocal tones, instrumental patterns of harmonics, and the traditional word-of-power theory. These are often indicated in our examples and text, but an extended study of their application must be left for a future book.

Closely connected to the throat centre and the energized utterance of tones, is the ancient concept of the 'word of power'. No genuine magical or spiritually enlightening system will ever claim to possess 'words of power' that are superior, secret or in some way better than those of another religion, cult or belief. Any such suggestion is derived from ignorance or credulity, or even from wilful misdirection. What is found within genuine transformative systems or Mysteries is the means to activate energize and transmit traditional Words or Names in a manner that brings out their inherent but usually inactive spiritual meaning. Much of the meaning comes from initiatory experience or contemplation and inner realization, but the *vocal utterance* is a quite unique ability that relies upon activation of the throat centre.

If we take an example, that of a traditional word of power known in many forms worldwide, it will help to demonstrate the theory and practice. If this word is further activated by musical or pitched resonance, it can become a very potent vehicle or sonic symbol.

The word is an ancient Name, ascribed to the great source of all Being, the Mother Deep. In the West it is the name of the primal Goddess, and carries through into the Christian concept of the Virgin. In the East it is the resonance used to define the Void beyond the manifest Universe. The word is AMA. In this first form, the first of Three, it means the Dark Mother Deep, or Primal Ocean. It is not merely spoken, but chanted in a long resonant humming, and is particularly powerful for opening out the two power centres of the Earth and the Moon, our first and second centres corresponding to the feet and the genitals.

During our practice sessions with the basic four-note power centre system, this name can be added to the chant with great effect.

The name is not merely an intellectual attribute, nor a word derived from tradition without a rich inner meaning. In simple (but not ignorant or trivial) terms, we can recognize it as the type of sound uttered by infants to their mother, but this is no mere psychological label to pin upon the origin of the Word. It is a wonderful and mysterious phenomenon that is expressed in a myriad of voices. If we take the trouble to separate the Word into its Three Letters, we can look further within.

A is a sound of *opening*. It carries the Primal Breath, and the first uttered tone. It is, metaphysically, our nearest equivalent to the first Two stages of divine utterance — the Breath and the Tone that began all Being. It is an open-ended sound, one of the vowels that make language meaningful; vowels which are traditionally equated with the Spirit (Breath) in all magical alphabets.

M is a resonant sound of *bridging* or *carrying*. If the first sound of opening is continued but with closed lips, it becomes a humming. The shape of the letter 'M' is a glyph that reminds us of a Wave, and it is the universal vibration that sums up all individualized sounds into one comprehensive resonance.

The first two letters, therefore, A+M, mean that the primal utterance is carried forward, from the Unknown towards the Known, by a bridging or mediating power. In simple language, the Spirit moves upon the face of the Deep.[3]

Our third letter is A repeated; it represents an opening out of the inner power, from the Unknown by a wave, to the Known. The first *A* is *originative*, the *M* is mediating, the second *A* is *creative*. It is the spirit appearing in a new world. We can show this in a simple glyph (Fig.

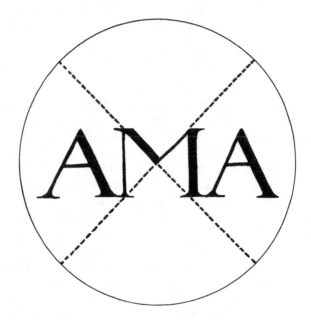

Fig. 17 A Universal Tone Word

17). Significantly, the Word AMA can be uttered in either direction, from the Unknown to the Known, or from the Known to the Unknown. The bridging tone of M flows either way. For us it acts as resonance that attunes our consciousness to inner reality, while for the source of creation, it acts as a medium whereby energy flows out to generate the outer and ultimately the material worlds.

The Word, as we discovered, is the magical equivalent of the Spirit moving on the face of the Deep, and at first it moves in a dimension that seems, to us, to be without light. It is the Dark Primal Mother.

This Word, therefore, will attune to the two lower power centres, which are of the nature of Earth and Water. If it is uttered with an activated throat centre, it can work to stir and enliven not only our own centres, which are also brought alive through our own imagination and discipline, but to resonate to the centres of other people. It also resonates through the metaphysical worlds, and can be heard in many different dimensions.

To carry this Word further, we need to examine the Second aspect of the Name, in which we add a further letter. By doing so, we symbolize the Dark Mother Filled with Light, and this is uttered by inserting an *I* into the word. The result is the Name: AIMA.

The effect of this new vowel is considerable; it stands for *Light*, or in the elemental world for *Fire*. As a glyph the letter *I* represents the Rod, the magical implement of power; the straight line; the male polarity. There is also an element of word-play, for in magical symbolism words often relate to one another in quite complex ways.[4] We can easily make the connections between *I*, the letter, 'I' the individuality, and the Eye that sees the Light. This apparently superficial type of connection produces remarkable results in meditation, and should not be reduced to mere psychological terms of association. The connectives must be pushed very deeply into the consciousness, until they are realized at a primal level during wordless contemplation.

By inserting this new vowel sound, our Word or chant now mirrors the appearance of the Light within the Depths, and we find that it appears *before* the bridging resonance of the M. The Word now names the Dark Mother, and restates the inner truth of the appearance of Light in the Primal Deep; this Light is carried out into the outer worlds by the Bridge (M) Resonance, where it is manifest in the form of the second *A*, the Mother of Natural Creation, which to us is the material world and its life forms, including of course ourselves.

We are not concerned, for the present, with the forms taken by this symbolism in other worlds, as we are dealing exclusively with the resonant effect of musical and magical words upon human power centres.[5]

As this second aspect of the Name now has the element of Light and Fire within it, it corresponds to our third power centre, that of the heart. Thus when raising the pitch and attuning the centres, we also insert the magically charged vowel into the chant: AMA/AIMA.

The third aspect of the Name is the form used as a word of power worldwide, both in Eastern and Western religion and meditative or magical practices. It consists of closing or summating the resonance of the second A with a final humming tone, the sound represented by our letter N. This gives us AIMAN, but it is usually pronounced AMEN or AUMEN. [6]

The second humming sound, N is thinner than the Bridging M, and a few brief experiments will prove that it pushes the sound upwards into the nose, actually making a resonance in the nose and upper sinus cavities. It is this region that is indicated for the power centre of the Forehead, and the physical resonance of the letter N (as a drawn out chant note) is a foreshadowing of the arousal of the power centre.

'AMEN' is traditionally the magical word of summation, used in orthodox Christianity merely to mean 'let it be so' or as a punctuation mark to group prayer. In esoteric usage, it is the word of Peace, of balanced power.

The closing N symbolizes (and stimulates) our understanding of creation moving into an entirely new dimension, by a balancing power that brings all energies to a peaceful union. In the working of the Inner Fire, it signifies an opened higher centre, a centre attuned to the mysterious but accessible higher modes of consciousness. [7]

9.

Vowel Sounds and Music

In our basic exercises and construction of the Musical Mirror, a basic *humming* expressed the tones or pitches that made up the music of the elemental psyche. We can now deal briefly with the ancient and important theory of vowel sounds in relationship to magic and spiritual psychology; before working on the material in this section familiarity and practice with the earlier exercises is essential, but both techniques are equally important and the use of vowel sounds is not 'more advanced' or 'important' than the primal resonance or humming sound.

Humming, the primal sound that *bridges* the First Breath (as in Chapter 8) is made with the mouth closed. A development, therefore, in human expression, is to open the mouth and so release vowel sounds. While this may appear to be a superficially obvious statement, the basic *closed* and *open* resonances of the voice are the roots of our vocal expression of inner energies, from the foundational emotions of early childhood to the sophisticated employment of intellectually loaded speech.

The basic rules of sound, music and the elemental psyche that harmonize with a transpersonal consciousness are so simple and direct that they have been ignored or forgotten in this century. Like the ubiquitous Philosopher's Stone they are so commonplace that no value is usually attached to them, while deluded seekers after spurious 'occult power' hunt high and low for secrets, and psychologists lose the trail in their obsession with labelling and reductionism. In Celtic fairy lore, one of the great secrets revealed to a mortal was that humans foolishly threw away the water with which they boiled their eggs; we might well suggest that this water is the primal or elemental psyche, shown in the traditional models employed here (but not in any way restricted to them, as they are open-ended and spiralling models of growth). We spend so much time upon the end-products of consciousness, the eggs, that we throw away the most important water that boiled them in the first place.

In the sound secret, this water is the humming sound, the closing bridging or menstruum consciousness that carries waves between the worlds.

The consciousness which employs music for inner or metaphysical operations is at once primal, simplistic and transcendent. Although models and open-ended systems are traditionally employed as clues to this consciousness and its effects, they are mere indicators; just as music cannot be taught through reading a book upon music, neither can metaphysics or magic be taught by studying the systems and maps or expressed alphabets. In both music and magic, however, the analogies drawn (the tutor book, the symbolic system) may give the questing mind a few handholds upon the real nature of the subject — which can only be *done* rather than *learned*.

Moving our musical model into the use of vowels, we must return to the basic statement that human emission of certain tones or sounds is a direct reflection of a cosmic universal creative emission of states of being, Worlds, or the physical and metaphysical consensus. This reflective and harmonic quality runs through all experiments with consciousness and cannot be divorced from them — hence many of the silly notions regarding magic and its inherent dangers. In our musical context, we are creating an elemental mirror of tones, pitches and shapes, which are directly harmonized by modes of consciousness within the human psyche and by energies within the greater universe.

Vowels are the core of vocal communication and as such were given a spiritual recognition and respect by early cultures. In some highly refined alphabets, such as that of Hebrew mysticism, vowels are sacred; they are the power tones of divinity and in one sense are direct aspects of that divinity. In a pantheistic system, vowels are not only archetypical powers, they are gods or goddesses in a most simple and primal state before more typified manifestation.

Consonants act as intersections between vowels, they make a framework upon which progressively complex orders of manifestation may grow. This is true both verbally and transcendentally; the Names of Power or of deities are cycles, rotations of intensely powerful vibrant vowels united with chosen consonants. When we apply this concept today we need not be mysterious, occult or even religious about the nature of vowels; such attitudes are valueless unless they reflect inner cognition and certainty. As intellectual elitist concepts the published theories on Words, Vowels and Names are in danger of becoming the inverse of their inner counterparts — empty theory with no enlivening spirit.

Traditionally a vowel is assigned for each Element and for the related attributes or cyclical harmonics of the Four Quarters as they rotate. For our present purpose we merely acknowledge that vowels are the undeniable heart and core of utterance. If there is any doubt about the truth of this statement, spend a few minutes trying to utter consonants without vowels; it simply cannot be done. Consonants cannot be uttered without vowels, but vowels can be uttered without consonants.

In the Elemental system a vowel is used to speak for and of a Quality (such as Air, Fire, Water or Earth) regardless of how that Quality manifests in various worlds. This cycle or spiral is found repeatedly in diagrams, glyphs and mandalas worldwide, reflecting a property or expression of human consciousness harmonizing and relating to the greater consciousness or the universe.

By using a vowel for each Quarter we are most emphatically not merely following orthodox religious use or occult teaching. We are going directly to the source of consciousness from which such usage derives. This source is nothing less than collective and individual intuition and meditation upon vowels and roots of communication through the Elements. Such meditations are extremely rewarding and productive in their own right, and will greatly benefit the practical use of the musical/metaphysical theories outlined in this book.

In music we are concerned first and foremost with the practical application of controlled sounds relating to the human psyche. To achieve this we can proceed directly to attribution of vowels to Elements without spending too much time in discussion of philosophical derivations. The actual physical resonance triggers the changes of consciousness. This cannot be stressed too often; most of the rest is mere verbiage or wilful obscurity on the part of writers, who wished to maintain orthodox superiority within a religion, church or esoteric organization. What is required of the practitioner is an honest effort to work with the symbols and maintain some basic simple disciplines; if you can do that, musical magic, metaphysics and the sound secret will come alive.

Sidestepping academic and linguistic research altogether, we can proceed to a practical allocation of vowels which may be used in chant or tonal utterance. The following cycle has been found to be very effective:

Air: Vowel Sound 'E' (pronounced as ee)
Fire: Vowel Sound 'I' (pronounced as long i)
Water: Vowel Sound 'O' (pronounced as long o)
Earth: Vowel Sound 'A' (pronounced aah)
Unity: Vowel Sound 'U' (pronounced long u or oo)

The last vowel sound 'U' is the synthesis of the Four Elements, expressing unity, truth or Spirit.

The further development of vowels as *visual* symbols is a very important magical matter which we cannot deal with here. Further attributes are found in our Appendix on *The Four Elements*.

Simplicity is all; the direct use of vowels is of far greater value than comparisons and historic origins. If we become bogged down in dispute or intellectual structures, the primal power is dissipated, and it is this primal power that we need to reinstate. Vowels are an unavoidable expression of our psychic-biological entity through sound; even our understanding of tone quality from instruments is expressed in terms that relate to the voice (vowels) or more confusedly, to colour.

Use of Vowels

In practice one vowel represents and utters one Element. From this first stage is developed the practice of vowels acting as powerful concentrated focii or matrices for all or any of the attributes of each Quarter. These attributes are suggested in Appendix 4.

Note: 'E'/Air/whistling/wind/arrow/cutting/sword/arising/dawn/east/morning/spring/beginning/freshness/youth/life/alertness/questing.

When we apply the vowels to elemental musical tones, the entire relationship begins to come alive. Magical harmonics or attributes are far more potent than the modern concept of 'word play' or 'free association'. The amalgams of consciousness or related symbol groups are impersonal and highly charged with potential energy to transform and vitalize the individual or group psyche. Hence the superstitious nonsense which surrounds words of power.

The basic steps of use are as follows:

1. Gain some experience in relating the vowels to the Elements. This may be done by rotating the elemental concepts upon a constant pitch or note, while changing the vowels with each cycle of the Elements. (i.e.: *chant* E/I/O/A/U/ *hum*. This sequence symbolizes and vitalizes Air/Fire/Water/Earth/Spirit/*consciousness*.)

2. Return to the Elemental calls which are demonstrated in our musical experiment constructing the Mirror. Each of these may be chanted or sung with its appropriate vowel. The call for Air (CFDE) would therefore be uttered with an *Eee* sound, Fire with an *Iii* sound, Water an *Oh* sound, and Earth an *Ah* sound. These should be smooth, elongated and continuous sounds, not broken or segmented.

One of the most ancient methods of such chanting is to *elide* or smoothly run the notes together, sliding up and down the intervals in a fully 'chromatic' sense. This is hardly ever done in modern art or commercial music, but is found still in some of the decorative styles of ethnic music worldwide. Metaphysically it is the full spectrum between each defined note that holds the power, while the notes themselves (CDEF, etc.) are merely points of definition. As music became increasingly formalized and rigid, this old magical technique was restricted and eventually passed out of common use altogether. If this curious method of chanting is too strange or difficult to the modern mind and voice, we can use the basic defined notes with almost equal effect, and under some circumstances (such as specific tone quality, melody shape, or harmony) with more effect.

The Elemental calls can be enhanced considerably by the incorporation (or inspiration) of vowels; the vowels cause a deep response in our organism, both physically and psychically, though it is not usual to be consciously aware of this effect. By employing the exercises and musical concepts, Hermetic musicology, we find ways to heighten our consciousness of the effect of music upon our entities.

If we add the development of controlled symbols (the attributes of the Elemental Quarters) and a willed use of the imagination, the organic and psychic response is further amplified.

There are, therefore, three distinct aspects of utterance for the music of an elemental psyche (metaphysical or magical music):

1. musical tones (defined points or levels of pitch vibration);
2. musical shapes (defined relationships between selected vibrations of differing rates);
3. musical vowels (defined primary expressions of consciousness as tonal *qualities* rather than vibrational *quantities*).

These are all, incidentally, found within the primal humming sound.

With some work, we are able to reduce lengthy and dull lists and series of symbolic correspondences to a small number of musical calls or sonic glyphs. These work with great rapidity in serial time, for they express consciousness that would otherwise be dulled by voluminous literary attributes, the bane of nineteenth and twentieth century 'occultism'.

A working meditator, magician or tonal therapist should not, in fact, need to think in terms of 'correspondences' at all, other than in the earliest stages of introductory training. He or she utters concentrated tones or shapes which *of themselves* generate and enhance all the attributes by stating their primary source and power. This root power, expressed in a unified fourfold spiralling model, causes changes in the outer world, which is firstly the consciousness and body of the person chanting or playing, then that of the listener or of other entities or objects which can resonate to the vibrations emitted.

This use of primal powers is quite alien to the modern mind, which is strongly conditioned to think that wholes are made only from an assembly of many parts — be they motor car parts or atomic particles. In the alternative modes of consciousness, expressed by ancient metaphysics and magic, parts are merely hologramatic representations of a diminishing series of wholes; or conversely, parts are the devolving cycle of a unity that exists in a higher order or reality. All parts ultimately partake of one whole.

In our musical work, the sound secret, human consciousness approaches wholeness by a number of very simple music utterances . . . the most simple basics of the musical scale and its cycle of partials. By this means, all spiralling creation may be attuned to one note, or four shapes, and given a voice through a few vowel sounds.

Appendix 1.

A Musical Diet

Some general notes on music in changing consciousness:

1. *Always be selective in your music.* Do not merely accept whatever is generated by the television, radio or musical plumbing of your home, work or social gathering place. Such selectivity becomes increasingly difficult in modern society, but you should not be afraid of making a nuisance of yourself; if music in a restaurant or shop is too loud, ask the staff to turn it down. Most people merely accept musical pollution, and never think of attempting to control it. Do not succumb to this attitude.

2. *Musical consciousness begins at home.* Do not have the radio or television on 'for company'. To truly relate to music you should listen to it as fully as possible, or not listen to it at all. Most media output works upon consciousness through our failure to truly *listen*. Regard a period of music-free time in the same way as you might consider a change of diet or a healthy fast: you are clearing out poisons from your system, and when this is done successfully you feel fitter, brighter and more aware.

3. *Avoid high-volume music,* particularly in rock or pop concerts, or in discotheques. This rule must also apply to music played at home, or at social gatherings; if the music is loud and you cannot control it, merely retire to some spot where it is less prevalent. Sheer volume acts as a drug, triggering our power centres in devolved or unhealthy ways, while certain combinations of rhythm, lights and bass frequencies are known medically to produce imbalance, physical illness and, in extreme cases, fits. After a period of 'music fasting', you will be amazed at how potent the effect of orchestral music can be, while you may well be nauseated by a trip to the local night-spot. This is not a matter of snobbery or elitism, but of mechanics, biology and psychology. In all fairness we must add that certain classical and avant garde musical forms can be most depressing and unhealthy.[1]

4. *Develop a taste for primal music.* This may be difficult at first, particularly if you are conditioned to commercial product or to strictly classical music. A number of recordings are listed in the Discography, and these might form the basis for further exploration into primal music. Once again, primal music triggers certain primal areas of our consciousness, and we cannot truly expect to appreciate the magic of music unless we are in contact with these vital areas within ourselves.

5. *Practise chanting or humming to yourself.* Not long ago people sang often; nowadays we hardly sing at all, unless we are copying a current hit song. Do not be put off by any subjective worry about whether your singing is 'good' or not; it is the act of making musical sound with your voice that is important, not a public concert. The chanting and resonating humming may be combined with meditation, as set out in our exercises, or they may merely be a daily effort to use the voice musically. Both extremes are equally important for our musical health.

6. *Use your own voice; do not mimic popular accents.* There is a very widespread habit of mimicking the accents used in product music songs. Do not do this; be prepared and willing to use your own natural voice, for that is your best sound. In some of us the habit of singing in bizarre accents is deeply ingrained, and the use of a cassette tape recorder may be a helpful corrective.

7. *Try to learn a musical instrument.* Once again, professionalism is quite irrelevant, for it is the act of making music that is of magical or spiritual significance, not the fashionable opinion or standard of that music.

Instead of merely doing exercises or simple pieces, try playing single notes in repetition, or listening to the instrument with your entire attention on each single sound that it makes. According to the metaphysical traditions, every time you cause a note to occur, you are mirroring the creation of the universe

8. *Spend a daily period of time in total silence.* This is a most important type of meditation, and need only last 10-15 minutes. A regular habit or a silent period each day will transform your response to all kinds of music within a relatively short period of time (after about one month).

9. *Listen to music under meditative circumstances.* Sitting with eyes closed in a room without disturbance, play some music on a tape or disc. You will find that some types of music have a powerful inner effect upon you, while others that seem superficially attractive during compulsive social activity have little or no effect, or may even be offensive to a calm mind and body.

Appendix 2.

Ancient European Music

Much of our current impoverished musical state is due to a fallacy. The viewpoint that music has evolved over a number of centuries, and that it will continue to progress into the future. This fallacy is tantamount to equating music with technology rather than with humanity, as if better machines will enable us to be better occupants of the planet Earth.

There can be little doubt that music has changed, quite radically, since the days of classical Greece, but we are too prone to assume that our music is more complex than that of the ancients. The true picture is one of cycles or spirals, much like the musical vibrations themselves which open outwards forever — except in our European art music where they are artificially contained in circles.

If we listen to recordings of traditional music, we are immediately plunged into music of enormous complexity, both in style, rhythm, and in the type and quality of modes and scales employed. This subtlety runs directly counter to the majority of theories published about musical development, in which folk music is often passed off as simple and boorish, or perhaps a crude copy of liturgical music or other musical styles. Sadly, very few musicologists or classical musicians ever listen to European traditional music; some even reach out to the East for inspiration, failing to find the subtlety in their own backyards. Like the alchemical stone, traditional music is a source of enormous wealth that is found everywhere but ignored by almost everyone.

The music of ancient Western cultures, therefore, should not be dismissed as inferior, merely because time separates us from it and we tend to equate time with evolution.

The Greeks made some very definite comments upon music, which have been handed down to us in corrupt form, implying that music contained certain well-defined powers over the consciousness. If we apply these comments today, and find that they do not make sense, we tend to shrug off the ancient theories as irrelevant due to evolution or to mere ignorance on the part of their originators.

There are a number of famous classical statements about music which are worth considering briefly in our context of music and changing consciousness. Although our own consciousness has materialized and externalized in certain collective mechanistic directions (passed off as individualism), we still hold within us the seeds of awareness that were held in common by early cultures. To test this theory, we must discover if early musical experiments or commentaries upon consciousness may still be effective, but this effect cannot be expected to apply immediately to our daily outward lives, so different from those of our ancestors. As mentioned in an earlier chapter we should not attempt to ape the past, but to bring the best of the past out into the present, ready for transformation towards the future.

Music has a tendency to home in to certain reiterations, patterns and relationships. We may find that the music of the future is a new cycle of the music of the past, a higher octave upon the spiral of time consciousness and sound.

1. **Plato.** *Republic* III. The origin of many repeated ideas on music in education or proper development of culture. Certain modes, rhythms, and even instruments, were banned by Plato, while others were acceptable. The judgement was based upon their effects within the listener. Regardless of the specific modes cited, the theory still has much validity; we know that music in early life has lasting effects upon the development of the psyche; the mass effect of music upon crowds is as commonplace today as it was in earlier cultures.

2. **Aristotle.** *Politics* VIII. Music in education for virtue, leisure and intellectual entertainment. Aristotle repeats the theory that music affects human character, suggesting that certain modes and instruments should be banned.

3. **St Augustine.** *Confessions* X, 33. Advises that the 'affectations of our spirit' correspond to certain musical modes. He also defines music as 'skilled movement which causes delight within itself' (*De Musica*).

4. **Boethius.** *De Musica.* The most important work widely used by medieval and later scholars. Was essential to musical degree studies in Oxford right up to the middle of the nineteenth century. Written in the sixth century this book describes many of the technical problems of acoustics and music with clarity and accuracy; the author claims

Pythagoras as his source and authority. Boethius clearly demonstrates the matter of Intonation (the problem of varying frequencies in nature which eventually led to the compromise of temperament. Related to the spiral of expanding fifth intervals described in our main text).

In Book 1, chapter 1, Boethius connects music with morality and quotes Plato (perhaps from memory or a source now lost) as saying that the behaviour of a republic can have no greater stain than to abandon upright and honourable music.

5. **Thomas Aquinas**. *Summa* and other works. Made many interesting comments and analyses of music, often drawn from sources such as the above listed. Musical proportions as intervals; acoustic experiments with weights; and a reiteration of the psychological power of certain modes or scales are typical of the subjects covered. A change of mode will change a mood as in Boethius' traditional tale ascribed to Pythagoras: a young man inflamed with drink (or lust) was stopped from burning his friend's house (or entering a brothel) by Pythagoras' instructions to a nearby musician. The musician changed the mode (note pattern) in which he played, and the young man's ardour was softened immediately.

Moving away from Aquinas we find this theme repeated in the *Vita Merlini* of Geoffrey of Monmouth (twelfth century). Merlin is insane and running wild in the woods; he is coaxed back to civilization by the music of a *cithara* (probably a *crwth* in this Welsh Celtic context, an instrument similar to a simple lyre played with a bow).

The Myth of Er

It is generally assumed that systems of musical metaphysics are all detailed from Plato and Pythagoras. If we adopt a literary and historical point of view, this seems self-evident; Plato is the earliest source, in written form, of such material, from whom subsequent philosophers and metaphysicians drew.

The classical example is the famous Myth of Er, from Plato's *Republic*, which includes a specific musical cosmology, related to both astrology and acoustics. The significance of this model, however, is greater than that of an authoritative or primary source. As we have suggested, such models arise within human consciousness; they are the spontaneous result of attempts to perceive 'reality' or 'truth' in a musically reflective pattern. This, in turn, is one expression of metaphysics, rooted to a physical acoustic ground in our outer world.

The vision described in Plato's story of Er is a timeless and operable one. We may experience it and use it ourselves. The literary complexity of the text is the result of reducing the vision to mere words; it is rendered more complex by this means. The system suggested in Chapter 5 is a simplified variant of the vision of Er.

Despite this close relationship, our original diagrams are not derived from the Platonic text, as they were assembled several years before the myth of Er was drawn to my attention. The similarities are, as a musical alchemist might say, harmonic: both visions and musical systems derive from a true Archetype, the celestial or primal music that is perceived only by inner direction, in meditation or inspired psychic ferment. Musical and magical systems are so consistent in this respect; they are harmonically attuned to a mode of perception, a reflection of Truth, and although they differ over words and technical details, they harmonize in their conceptual patterns.

In other words, similarities between musical systems do not necessarily imply literary progression or inheritance. They indicate a certain unity between human beings that cuts through both time and space to create our impressions of the Music of the Spheres.

He also added, that every one, after they had been seven days in the meadow, arising thence, it was requisite for them to depart on the eighth day, and arrive at another place on the fourth day after, whence they perceived from above through the whole heaven and earth, a light extended as a pillar, mostly resembling the rainbow, but more splendid and pure; at which they arrived in one day's journey; and they perceived, being in the middle of the light from heaven, that its extremities were fastened to the sky. For this light was the belt of heaven, like the transverse beams of ships, and kept the whole circumference united. To the extremities the distaff of Necessity is fastened, by which all the revolutions of the world were made, and its spindle and point were both of adamant, but its whirl mixed of this and of other things; and that the nature of the whirl was of such a kind, as to its figure, as is any one we see here. But you must conceive it, from what he said, to be of such a kind as this: as if in some great hollow whirl, carved throughout, there was such another, but lesser, within it, adapted to it, like casks fitted one within another; and in the same manner a third, and a fourth, and four others, for that the whirls were eight in all, as circles one within another, each having its rim appearing above the next; the whole forming round the spindle the united solidity of one whirl. The spindle was driven through the middle of the eight; and the first and outmost whirl had the widest circumference, the sixth had the next greatest width; the fourth the third width; then the eighth; the seventh; the fifth; and the second. Likewise the circle of the largest is variegated in colour; the seventh is the brightest, and that of the eighth hath its colour from the shining of the seventh; that of the second and fifth resemble each other, but are more yellow than the rest. But the third hath the whitest colour, the fourth is reddish; the second in whiteness surpasses the sixth. The distaff must turn round in a circle with the whole it carries; and whilst the whole is turning round, the seven inner circles are gently turned round in a contrary direction to the whole. Again, the eighth moves the swiftest; and next to it, and equal to one another, the seventh, the sixth, and the fifth; and the third went in a motion which as appeared to them completed its circle in the same way as the fourth, which in swiftness was the third, and the fifth was the second in speed. The distaff was turned round on the knees of Necessity. And on each of its circles there was seated a Siren on the upper side, carried round, and uttering one note in one tone. But that the whole of them, being eight, composed one harmony. There were other three sitting round at equal distances one from another, each on a throne, the daughters of Necessity, the Fates, in white vestments, and having crowns on their heads; Lachesis, and Clotho, and Atropos, singing to the harmony of the Sirens; Lachesis singing the past, Clotho the present, and Atropos the future. And Clotho, at certain intervals, with her right hand laid hold of the spindle, and along with her mother turned about the outer circle. And Atropos, in like manner, turned the inner ones with her left hand. And Lachesis touched both of these, severally, with either hand. Now after the souls arrive here, it is necessary for them to go directly to Lachesis, and then an herald first of all ranges them in order, and afterwards taking the lots, and the models of lives, from the knees of Lachesis, and ascending a lofty tribunal, he says: 'The speech of the virgin Lachesis, the daughter of Necessity. Souls of a day! This is the beginning of another period of men of mortal race. Your destiny shall not be given you by lot, but you should choose it yourselves. He who draws the first, let him first make choice of a life, to which he must of necessity adhere. Virtue is independent, which every one shall partake of, more or less, according as he honours or dishonours her. The cause is in him who makes the choice, and God is blameless!' When he had said these things, he threw on all of them the lots, and that each took up the one which fell beside him, but Er was allowed to take none. And that when each had taken it, he knew what number he had drawn.

Pythagoras and the Four Smiths

Our introductory poem at the beginning of the book is inspired by a number of alchemical illustrations and texts, in which Pythagoras is said to have discovered certain musical principles of both earthly and cosmic relationship, through a visit to a forge.

The source for this legend is Nicomachus of Gerasa (first — second centuries). His *Manual of Harmonics* describes the Pythagorean experience in detail, and to the informed reader it seems to be a visionary or even formal initiatory sequence:

He happened by good luck to pass by a blacksmith's shop, where he heard clearly the iron hammers striking the anvil and confusedly uttering sounds which gave, all but one, intervals of perfect consonance. . . . Thrilled he entered the workshop as if a god was aiding his plans, and after certain experiments he found that it was the difference of weights that caused the differences of pitch, and not the effort of the smiths, nor the shape of the hammers, nor the movement of the work.

Although this extract seems to be physically inaccurate, for hammer weights do not necessarily affect resonances from the objects under the hammer-action, it conceals a mystical and alchemical truth. Various scholars have theorized upon the nature of the Smith's work but it is obvious that if the sounds were uttered by the *metal under the hammer,* by the work itself, as in the keys or plates of a xylophone or glockenspiel, then weight does indeed cause differences of pitch. As Nichomachus also tells us that; 'With the greatest of care he [Pythagoras] measured the weights of the hammers and their impulsive force, which he found to be perfectly identical, then he returned home,' we can assert that the Pythagorean experiment is accurate. The remainder of Nichomachus' text is concerned with mathematical and acoustic formulae.

If we restore the initiatory vision according to the very simple Elemental principles described in our earlier text and diagrams, the result can be expressed as a verse. The subject of the work, that which emits a cycle of harmonics, the Fourfold Nature, is revealed to be human consciousness; yet paradoxically it is also the material world, the Four Elements.

Appendix 3.

Hermetic Music and Practices/Origin of Term 'Hermetic'

The prominent feature of Hermetic philosophy is not merely its historically ancient derivation but its method. Hermetic philosophy takes a group of conceptual models which have certain links, and intentionally merges them together to form new entities. This process is represented frequently by the alchemical experiment. To the student of higher consciousness, esoteric symbolism, or even modern psychology (to a limited extent) it is known that conceptual models arise from the action of consciousness reflecting upon the properties of space, time and energy — the univerise.

In Hermetic music, or magical music, or primal music, we meet this facility at work. At one extreme we have sophisticated symbol systems (as in Fludd, Kircher, or Maier) while at the other we have the sacred-magical utterance of tones impelled by a driving consciousness attuned to cycles of life such as the seasons or the positions of the stars. The only difference between the two extremes is the use of a written language and the associated structures of intellectual communication that writing generates. Otherwise they both say the same thing: *all life is linked by a spiral of harmonies.*

In alchemical work, bio-electrical energies (such as those known to exist in interchanges of polarity from sexual activity through to meditation), are applied to minerals. This is an example of following a conceptual model through to the point where its boundaries dissolve and it merges with another model. In music, our psychic and physical responses are partly generated through the application of simple laws of acoustics; these in turn connect to mathematics, which leads to astronomy, then onwards around the spiral to modern atomic physics.

It is easy, therefore, to swim in the Hermetic ocean of dissolution, but quite difficult to pull out any fish! Conceptual models or patterns (be they mathematical or magical) are specific crystallizations out of a solution of general consciousness-in-being; this consciousness is an impressionable medium receiving signals from various orders of existence, then mediating these signals (polarity exchanges of energy) for specifically limited purposes. It is valueless to swim in the liquid area where sets of concepts merge, and then blandly suggest that 'all is one'. This is the great weakness of the modern revival of music, magic and metaphysics, in terms of a so-called New Age.

The Hermetic process dissolves sets of concepts as chemicals are dissolved in a solution; at a certain moment crystals are formed within this solution, and their pattern is brought back into expression as new models, systems or symbols expressed in complex language. The language is not the crystal itself, but leads the student to repeat the experiment with some chance of success.

Scientific discoveries are often made through intuitive leaps across conceptual boundaries, which are later confirmed by material experimentation. Hermetic science, which is also an art, sets out the means whereby the leaps may be made, and music, in a very specific sense, is one such means.

It is the urge to bridge across sets of symbols or to link arts and sciences that has led to the advance of modern materialist thought; yet this urge is deeply mystical, and paradoxically the advance of science has led into further specialization to the point of fragmentation and on to alienation. If we attempt to concentrate this bridging quality in a specific study of music and the psyche, we rapidly find a set of transformative symbols (the tones and the Elemental calls) that swim hidden in the depths of the musical ocean, yet are an essential part of its life-cycle.

A truly Hermetic approach to music, therefore, is not one of listing works of music or musical evolutionary phases, but one of boiling all music down to potent and original units. In Celtic legend this was the Cauldron of the UnderWorld in which magical power, foresight and regeneration were to be found.

Origin of the Term 'Hermetic'

This popular term, much beloved by the alchemists, is a catch-all for the wisdom of the ancient cultures. *Hermes-Trismegistus* (Thrice Great) was a mythical person, and many works were ascribed to him, mainly those of Egyptian Neo-Platonists.

The Egyptian god Thoth, the Intellect, was identified by the Greeks with their own Hermes at least as early as the time of Plato (*c.* 400 BC). In the struggle between Neo-Platonism and Christianity, the ancient authority of both Egypt and Greece was combined by the Neo-Platonists, taking up a tradition that runs through cultures worldwide, that of the semi-divine origins of human knowledge. Thoth-Hermes was cited as the source of all inventions and secret wisdom, from whom Pythagoras and Plato drew their ideas. In other words, they drew upon Mystery traditions and artistic sciences rooted in the cultural development of the Western world.

Clement of Alexandria (second to third centuries) mentions 42 books of Hermes extant in his day; Iamblichus (fourth century) mentions 20,000 while Manetho (third century BC) is supposed to have cited 36,525 such books. These rather uncertain figures merely represent a typical tradition of extensive knowledge.

By the thirteenth century, the Hermetic tradition had been taken up by the alchemists, who expanded it and refined their own variants of it. *The Precepts of Hermes* (see Read 1961) translated from an early source (possibly Greek) through a number of languages and texts, were said to be the embodiment of the *Hermetic* art in a concentrated form. Many of the precepts bear a similarity to mystical, magical and related musical concepts.

The Emerald Table (Precepts of Hermes)

1. I speak not of fictitious things, but that which is certain and true.
2. What is below is like that which is above, and what is above is like that which is below to accomplish the miracles of unity.
3. As all things were produced by the one word of one Being, so all things were produced from this one thing by adaptation.
4. Its father is the sun, its mother the moon, the wind carries it in its belly, its nurse is the earth.
5. It is the origin of perfection throughout the world.
6. The power is vigorous if it be changed into earth.
7. Separate the earth from the fire, the subtle from the gross, acting with prudence and judgement.
8. Ascend with the greatest wisdom from earth to heaven, and then descend again to earth and unite together the powers of things superior and things inferior. Thus will you obtain the glory of the whole world and obscurity will fly far away from you.
9. This has more fortitude than fortitude itself; because it conquers every subtle thing and can penetrate every solid.
10. Thus was the world formed.
11. Hence proceed wonders which are here established.

12. Therefore I am called Hermes Trismegistos, having three parts of the philosophy of the whole world.
13. That which I have said today concerning the operation of the sun is now complete.

Appendix 4.

The Four Elements

Air: Beginning/Birth/Inception/First Breath/
Dawn/Morning/Childhood/Sunrise/
Thinking/Questioning/Emerging/Arising/
Sword/Arrow/Cutting/Flying/Moving/
Liberty/Leaping/Exciting/*Life*/
Wind/Fresh/Power/Sound/
Spring/Germination/Inspiration/Attention.
Vowel sound: E.

Fire: Increasing/Adulthood/Continuing/Exhalation/
Noon/Brightness/Ability/Zenith/
Directing/Controlling/Incandescent/Burning/
Rod/Ruling/Balancing/Upright/
Seeing/Relating/Harmonizing/*Light*/
Flame/Heat/Energy/Colour/
Summer/Growth/Illumination/Perception.
Vowel sound: I

Water: Fulfilling/Maturity/Culminating/Second Breath/
Evening/Ending/Fullness/Sunset/
Feeling/Receiving/Settling/Flowing/
Cup/Giving/Purifying/Sustaining/
Nourishing/Cleansing/Clarifying/Emotion/*Love*/
Autumn/Harvest/Sharing/Intuition.
Vowel sound: O.

Earth: Ceasing/Age/Rest/Exhalation/
Night/Darkness/Peace/Starlight/
Supporting/Reflecting/Solidify/Manifesting/
Shield/Mirror/Returning/Grace/

Coldness/Dryness/Containment/Touch/*Law*/
Winter/Waiting/Preserving/Expression.
Vowel sound: A.

(Many more attributes may be added to these sequences; the four interactions listed above are merely an indication of some of the major and traditional expressions of the Four Elements.)

Appendix 5.

Three Systems of Metaphysical Music

Having presented a very specific system of music for inner transformation, three further systems are shown here briefly for comparison. A large selection of such material with invaluable notes is found in Godwin (1986), a source book of references and systems for music and changing consciousness, taken from the range of literary sources available.

Three Comparable Systems

1. *The Proportional Tree of Life* (Fig. 18).
2. *The Sympathetic Harmony of the World*: one of the traditional musical/metaphysical systems adapted by Athanasius Kircher in his *Musurgia Universalis* (1650).
3. *The Magic Circle Maze Dance*: musical symbolism in a modern text by Gareth Knight (*The Rose Cross and the Goddess*, 1985).

The Proportional Tree of Life
Musical notes are frequently shown upon the Tree of Life in ascending and descending order, but as we have seen from our main text, music and the primal energies work in spirals, from which the selected pattern of the Tree, Tetractys, Elements, Zodiac and magical circle are derived.

The proportions of the scale (first, second, third and so on) are strict mathematical acoustic entities (except in modern music where they have been adjusted or tempered) and may be set upon the polarity pattern of the Tree of Life accordingly. In this system the notes 'ascend' and 'descend' simultaneously, and a number of sub-patterns are found by tracing the sequences around the Paths between the Spheres. Examples are given below (see also Fig. 18).

Spheres 10/9/8/6/7/9/10. Scale: CDEFGABC. The lower harmonic or

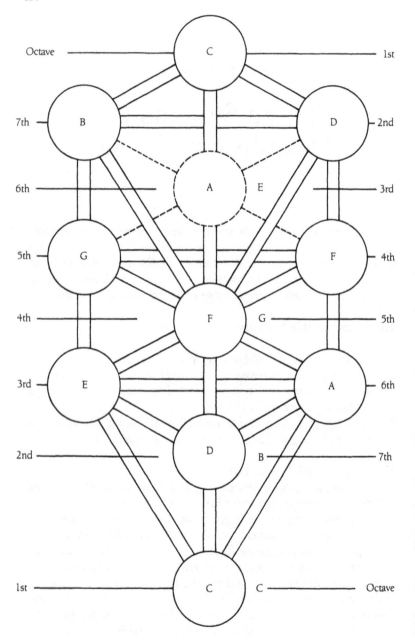

Fig. 18 The Proportional Tree of Life

lower five spheres of the Tree (Earth, Moon, Sun, Mercury and Venus) make a whole scale or 'world'. This is music (and reality) as we usually perceive it. It cycles from: 10 physical expression to: 9 biological response to: 8 intellectual response to: 6 harmony or spiritual response to: 7 emotional response to: 9 effect upon overall psyche and body; back to 10. (Kingdom to Foundation to Glory to Beauty to Victory to Foundation to Kingdom.) (See Fig. 3.)

This cycle is a very good way of showing what happens to the listener when he or she takes in and responds to a piece of music. If we follow the same notes around their progression through the upper Spheres, we find a harmonic relationship between this *life cycle of music* and the areas of consciousness that are not usually accessible to human beings:

C/C *The Kingdom and the Crown:* Spirit inherent in matter. 10/1 Octave.

C/D *Kingdom and Foundation:* links to B, *Understanding* 10/9+3. Musical intervals are the second and the seventh. (There is an understanding or intuitive consciousness inherent in the body and its life energies, or in matter and the stellar depths of space. The Lunar goddess, the Earth goddess, and the Great Mother, are part of one another.) The *second* and the *seventh* represent the *first* and *last* steps of our scale leading away from and back towards the octave.

C/E. *Kingdom and Glory:* Body and mind. 10/8. Interval of *third* links to note A, interval of *sixth*. (The intellect is a polarity of consciousness closely connected to the emotions, they react upon one another and so affect the body. Both notes (A+E, third and sixth of the scale) are found again at *Daath*, Knowledge/Experience, the Bridge over the Abyss between the Supernal or Upper Spheres and the remainder of the Tree of Life. The polar consciousness of the intellect and the emotions (spheres 8+7 Glory/Victory, Hermes/Venus) unites in a higher Knowledge that bridges the abyss between regular and transcendent cognition.) The *third* and the *sixth* are important proportions in music that define the *major* or *minor* quality of a work, scale, chord or melody. This quality generates a mental and emotional response within the listener.

E/F. *Glory and Beauty.* Mental activity attuned to spiritual or solar principles of Harmony. Spheres 8-6. Intervals of *third* and *fourth* from root note C. The *fourth* is one step beyond the responsive harmony of the *third*. This step is one *semitone* in size. (The intellect merges directly with a higher consciousness (Hermes and Apollo, Mercury and the Sun) which illuminates it and harmonizes its operation.)

The myth of Hermes making the Lyre for Apollo may be used here to show that the intellect or mental application or craft generates structures through which the inner power of Harmony or relationship or proportion may be expressed into the outer world. Once again we find a cosmic or higher expression in the relationship of the note E to *Daath* or the Bridging place over the Abyss: as Hermes is to Apollo (8/6, *Third* interval to *fourth* interval) so is the Bridge to the Crown. The *third* may also be a minor third, which gives one whole tone between third and fourth.

F/G. Represents the Triad of Power upon the Tree of Life, the 6th, 5th, and 4th Spheres: *Beauty, Severity and Mercy:* Sun, Mars, Jupiter. This is the cycle between the Power of Balance or the Source (6), the Power of Taking (5), and the Power of Giving (4). The intervals are the *fourth* and *fifth* from the *root note C* and have one tone between them.[1]

Returning to the step F/G, the Solar Triad has a number of important aspects in musics and metaphysics.

1. F/G is the transition between the upper and lower parts of the scale CDEF/GABC. As described in our main text, the upper part of the scale is a statement of the harmonics of the lower part, and vice versa. The central role of the Solar Triad shows this in its reiterative musical utterance; it is the heart of the music, and does not have any stated links to higher or lower notes as we can see from Fig. 18.

2. The Sixth Sphere (Tiphareth or Beauty) is the Solar and Harmonizing Sphere upon the Tree; it represents Balance, Illumination, Proportion, and the great images of salvation (Christ, Buddha) may be placed here in meditation. This Sphere has the notes F/G, the transition step, an interval of one tone place in the *middle* of the scale. The scale ascends in one direction and descends in another from this tonal location. The actual power of the Sixth Sphere is found exactly in the middle of that interval of one tone, a point which cannot be defined. The step from F to G contains within it partials or harmonics of all the other notes of the scale, deriving from that undefinable heart-location or seed source. This is the Crown, or first Sphere (Breathing Forth) within the Sixth Sphere (the Spirit within the Sons of Light in traditional terminology). In our individual consciousness it is the primal seed of being within the illuminated higher awareness that unifies the intellect and the emotions.

    We are rationalizing the symbols by using a basic scale of C major, but we may equally well use any locating note, and the principle of the middle or seed would still hold true.

3. The relationship is further expressed by the nature of the *fourth* and *fifth* intervals, for they are both 'equidistant' from our root note C

although different notes! F is one fourth (CDEF) above the lower C of a one octave C-C scale. It is also one fifth below the upper C of the same scale (FGABC). G is one fifth above the lower C (CDEFG) and one fourth below the upper C (GABC).

G and F, therefore, represent the polarizations (Spheres 4/5, or positive and negative, Mercy and Severity) of a resolving or unified bi-polar centre. (Sphere 6, Harmony, the combined tone G/F), or more specifically the mysterious source of that tone uttering both polar extremes simultaneously.

4. The step of one tone contains all other steps of the scale. This is not only true in acoustics, but is the basis for the unfolding of the Tree of Life and the Tetractys: 1+2+3+4=10.

In a tempered modern scale and in an untempered natural scale, we find that the tenfold progression is expressed by the chromatic intervals, between the notes C-F (which hold the *fifth* partials of G-C inherent within them). 1+2+3+4 gives us five semitones or C/Csharp/D/Eflat/E/F. Here is the much sought after resolution between the notes of music and the tenfold symbolism of the Tree of Life; this is a restatement of the Elemental theme of our main text, reduced to a proportional semitone sequence. If we divided it again into quarter-tones, we would have a Tree of Life plus its Paths, all expressed in increasingly chromatic or microtonal intervals. This becomes too minute for the modern ear and musical understanding, so it must be expanded to the larger spaces or intervals which we are accustomed to hearing.

Conclusions

The system outlined briefly above is perhaps the most advanced and flexible of any shown in this book. The reader can take it and add further harmonic connections by comparing the qualities and symbols of the Tree of Life with the musical connectives shown in Fig. 18. Our summary of the lower notes CDEFGABC or Spheres 10, 9, 8, 7, 6, covers the remainder of the Tree through the musical connectives.

The system of music and the power centres (Figs. 15 and 16) may be used with the musical notes shown in Fig. 18 for a further development of technique in chanting for meditation or psychic adjustment.

The Sympathetic Harmony of the World

Fr. Kircher's method of relating music to the Tree of Life follows a traditional format which he expands considerably. A summary of his system of the *Symphony of Nature in Ten Enneachords* is as follows:

Tone: 1st half, Angels/Earthly Elements/Sulphur/Lodestone/Wheat/
Fruits.

2nd half tone, Archangels/Moon/Silver/Crystal/Honesty (plant)/Pod
fruits.

Third: Principalities/Mercury/Quicksilver/Agate/Peony/Apple.

Fourth: Powers/Venus/Tin (usually copper)/Beryl/Orchid/Myrtle.

Fifth: Virtues/Sun/Gold/Garnet/Sunflower/Laurel.

Sixth: Dominions/Mars/Iron/Adamant/Absinthe/Oak.

Seventh: Thrones/Jupiter/Copper (usually tin)/Amethyst/Betony/
Lemon.

Octave: Cherubim/Saturn/Lead/Topax/Hellebore/Cypress.

Ninth: Seraphim/Firmament/Salt/Mineral stars/Stellar herbs/fruits.

Tenth: Deity/Empyrean.

The ten intervals relate to ten worlds which in turn correspond to the
Ten Spheres of the Tree of Life. Interval (1) the Tone is Sphere 10. As
copper and tin have been transposed so have Oak, usually ascribed to
Jupiter, and Lemon, with its astringent properties of Mars.

For a more detailed exposition see Godwin 1986, where a full table
is shown including attributes of animals, birds and colours.

The Magic Circle Maze Dance

(Extracted from Gareth Knight, *The Rose Cross and the Goddess*, 1985.[2]
Reproduced by permission of the author.)

Musical Symbolism

We can at this point introduce another mode of symbolic expression, that
of sound, for the circle and the cross can also be expressed in terms of
acoustics.

In the rituals of a certain Order, the Magus of the Lodge states that each
of the Officers represents 'a note in the chord of the ritual', and the Magus,
by contacting each officer, then proceeds 'to set that chord vibrating'.

That chord we may derive from the harmonics of a vibrating string. The
principles apply equally to a vibrating column of air, as in a wind instrument.
For the sake of simplicity we will confine our remarks to a string. This was
the device used by the Pythagorean philosophers to explain their
philosophical number system.

If a string is plucked, and set into vibration, it will emit a note. If we then
halve the length of the string, we find we have the 'same note', but at a higher
pitch. Similarly if we were able to double the length of the string the note
would again be 'the same', but at a lower pitch.

In the tonic solfa system, if our original note was *doh*, then halving the
string gives us *doh* at the top of the scale, and doubling it would give us
another *doh* at the bottom of the scale.

This is usually called being an 'octave' higher or lower. But to talk of octaves, or scales, is to assume too much at this point. The scale we are so accustomed to is but a local convention. Other civilizations have other scales which are just as valid. Indian, Chinese, Islamic, and European music sound different because they use different conventions. European music happens to use a scale of eight notes, hence the use of the term octave. This is not however a universal law. And even some European folk music uses a scale of six notes only.

The ancient Greeks were therefore more accurate in calling the space between the reappearance of a note at a lower or higher pitch as a 'diapason'. This distance in pitch, or diapason, can be divided into as many divisions as we choose. There are however certain natural divisions based on whole number divisions of a string. We have already discovered the importance of dividing or multiplying the string with the whole number 2.

By transforming a unity into an equal duality, we have created a diapason, an upper and a lower limit wherein a complete range of musical expression may be developed. This we can make the basis of another model universe, but in terms of sound rather than space.

We may now extend the model by introducing the number 3. If we take one third of the length of the string we strike a new note, that falls within the limits of the diapason. This new note differs from the fundamental note that defines the top and bottom of the diapason, yet it has an intimate feeling of relationship to it. It is, for this reason, in musical theory, called the 'dominant' note in the scale. The relationship should be experienced by the ear; it is the feeling of relatedness between *doh* and *soh* in the tonic solfa system. The whole of the Western system of musical keys is based upon this relationship between 'dominant' and 'tonic' note, and the 'cycle of fifths'.

This takes us into areas of musical theory which need not immediately concern us, although no time is wasted in acquiring the necessary technical knowledge to research further into this symbolism, which is intimately associated with the quality of numbers. The art and science of sonics is in fact the real basis of any system of numerology.

For our immediate purpose it is sufficient to say that the initial division of a string by whole numbers brings about particular fundamental soul experiences. And this forms the basic structure of a *musical* harmonic system, which may also be used to form the basis of a *magical* harmonic system.

Dividing a string by 2, we get the so-called octave, or the same note at a higher mode of manifestation. In tonic solfa this will be high *doh*.

Dividing the string by 3, we get the dominant note of any scale that one may choose to construct within the diapason of low and high *doh*. This is the so-called 'fifth', or tonic solfa *soh*.

If we divide the string by 4, we find a repetition of the tonic note at a yet higher arc; for a quarter is a half of a half, and we have introduced the principle of 2 again, in a different mode, or at a higher power (2×2 or 2^2). This would give us the higher *doh* above high *doh*.

If we divide the string into 5 we get another important note. This is generally called the 'third', or in the tonic solfa system, *me*. An important quality of this note is that it can manifest in one of two ways, each of which gives a different quality of feeling. In conventional musical terms this is called the major or minor mode. And, in very simplified terms, a piece of music will sound bright or sad according to whether the third note of the conventional scale is in the major or minor mode. (In the minor mode the 3rd is flattened.)

In symbolic terms of Pythagorean mathematics and musicology this dual mode of expression introduces the principle of polarity at a new level of expression. It is analogous to sexual and other expressions of polarity in manifestation.

Division by 6 need not detain us here. It is important philosophically in that it is a combination of the powers of the 2 and the 3. It will indeed produce a dominant note a whole scale higher. This is what might be expected from the principles of duality and triplicity combined. Harmonious expression on a higher arc.

We bring our investigation to a close by dividing the string by 7. This introduces a new quality that produces a note that is not found on our conventional scale. The principle of the number 7 throws out the balanced expression of the senarius (i.e., the numbers 1 to 6), and introduces a new quality that is outside the previously established conventions. These conventions, if they were to act alone, would simply produce ever repeating regular patterns. The 7 introduces a slightly jarring element into this infinite regular system and breaks it up into many possibilities of individual self-expression.

In musical terms the new note thus formed approximates to a flattened seventh, or a note midway between *lah* and *te* in the tonic solfa system. It does not have an entirely unpleasant sound, and may be found in natural expression in various forms of folk music.

In applying harmonic principles to the magical circle we select certain of these principal tones in much the same way that a bell is made to resonate to different harmonics of its fundamental strike tone through its shape and design. The magic circle might indeed be envisaged as a kind of psychic bell, that chimes forth at many inner levels.

In technical musical terms the four points of the circle may be described as making up a dominant seventh chord in the Dorian mode. To simplify and particularize this description: the East resounds forth the key note; the West the 'fifth' or dominant; the South the 'third' in its flattened mode; and the North the 'seventh', also in its flattened mode.

Thus if we make the keynote of the East the tone C: then the other notes are Eb in the South, G in the West, and Bb in the North. The flattened modes of South and North are chosen as being more natural. When skill is acquired in the use of this system, and appreciation of the subtlety of its possible extensions, then for particular occasions other modes may be used.

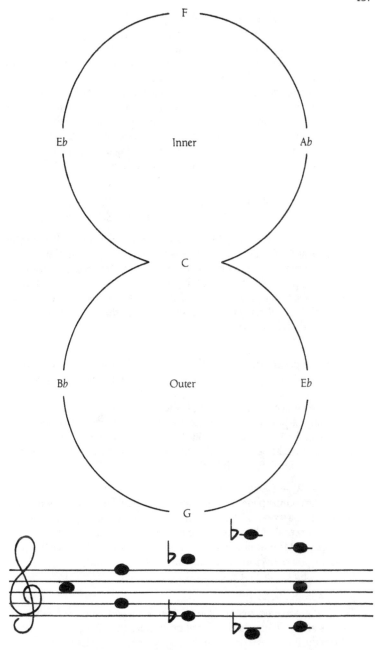

Fig. 19 Musical/Metaphysical Diagram by Gareth Knight

To keep matters simple, it is sufficient to associate the appropriate notes we have named with the appropriate quarters. This will provide a kind of musical magical shorthand. We can by these means encapsulate the principles of different ritual patterns by means of a short sequence of melody based on this magical harmonic structure.

It is on these principles that legends on the mighty effect of words of power are based. These basic facts are indeed the foundation on which may be reconstructed the art of mantic chanting. An art almost lost to the West but that has remained developed in the East, notably in Tibet.

Different ritual patterns may be described along lines that are similar to the way that a chime of bells is worked out, as a series of permutations. Thus:

C,	Eb,	G,	Bb,	C	E.	S.	W.	N.	E.
C,	Bb,	G,	Eb,	C	E.	N.	W.	S.	E.
C,	G,	Eb,	Bb,	C	E.	W.	S.	N.	E.

Note that in all of these combinations we are commencing and ending the sequence at the Eastern quarter. This is because it is from this Quarter that control is usually effected. Other combinations can be developed, using the centre as a point of control but the principles are best enunciated in the first instance by the patterns above. There is indeed considerable scope for further individual research and discovery once the basic principles are understood and experienced.

$E - S - W - N - E$

This is the pattern of circumambulation in a clockwise direction around the circle and is a way of raising power, particularly when there are participants seated around the circle contributing their psychic force by their presence and active participation in building, in the imagination, the images described. The rising of power can be conceived symbolically as the raising of the keynote of the East an octave at each circumambulation. This in melodic symbolism could be described as an upward movement of three octaves — C, Eb, G, Bb, C Eb G Bb C' Eb' Gb' C"

$E - N - W - S - E$

This is the counter pattern to the above, and useful for closing down power at the end of a working by anti-clockwise reverse circumambulations. The psychic power that has been raised is thus given back, enriched, to the participants. Melodically, this movement, with its inherent force flow and resultant power level in the circle, can be described as:
C" Bb' G' Eb C' Bb, G, Eb, C,

$E - W - S - N - E$

This is the general direction of force flow throughout the circle when the stations at the quarters are manned by responsible officers. Power comes in from the East by the principal of polarity line running East — West from the officer of the East, who is the link with the inner beings behind the working. It flows to the officer of the West who acts as a focus for the corporate entity of all present in the physical circle. The force then circulates round to the Officer of the South who mediates it in love to the rest of the group. In workings where there are just the three principal officers, as in those deriving from the Masonic pattern, the tradition is to have the neophytes seated opposite him in the North so that a particular force flow may be set up toward them. This may be assisted by a Novice Master seated with them in the North. From this point, which is the bottoming of the inner force, it returns to the Eastern office whence it originated. In its simplest expression this may be described in the melodic sequence C' G Eb Bb, C.

This would seem to represent a constant lowering of force but the method of working brings force through from the East and sets up higher harmonics from 'beyond the veil' so that what in effect happens is a general raising of levels. In practice, once the primary circuit is set up, the force will flow out from all officers; with its ultimate derivation being beyond the East on the inner, so that the whole pattern resembles a figure of 8; the Magus of the Lodge, in the East, being at the point joining the two circles of the inner and outer worlds.

The Magus thus forms a dominant to a higher key note on the inner. We may imagine that when the 'note' of the officer of the West is vibrating it stimulates the sounding of the Eastern Office of the inner Lodge. Then when the force proceeds to the Southern Officer and his note is sounded, a resonance is formed with the corresponding office on the inner; and likewise with the note of the Northern Office.

By these means a great chord is formed and the original key note is resonated at an upper and lower level from the original sounding.

Notes

1. Stewart 1985.
2. Scott 1958; Rudhyar 1982. Standard histories of music other than those with esoteric aims inevitably follow an 'evolutionary' theme.
3. Stewart 1986 (*Prophetic Vision of Merlin*).
4. The question of movement and direction is very relevant to music and changing consciousness; a straight line or generally linear movement, the popular concept of evolution, leads inevitably to the rigid unbending formalism of so-called classical music. Primal qualities of motion signify primal states of consciousness both individual and universal. 'The principal spiritual operations are described under an appearance of *position*. They are three differing movements, for example, *circular* whereby anything is moved uniformly round its centre; next *straight* according to which a thing proceeds from one to another; and the third *oblique* (a serpentine movement) which is made up of both circular and straight.' St Thomas Aquinas (my italics).
5. Rudhyar, 1982, 139-45.
6. Read 1961.
7. Gantz 1976; Knight 1978, 1983; MacCana 1975; Ross 1974; Rees, A and B (1961); Matthews 1986; Stewart 1976, 1981, 1985. All of the foregoing contain a wide cross-section of material demonstrating Western cultural and magical symbolism plus extensive references and bibliographies for further reading.
8. Chambers 1956 gives a number of important proofs of the origin of liturgical chant from folksong. Although his argument is concerned with early Christian plainchant, the proof of musical adaptation by the Church has significant links to the formal oral music of the pagan

religions. Many sophisticated systems of memorizing music were retained by Celtic peoples until at least the eighteenth century.

9. Stewart 1985; Matthews vols. 1 and 2 1985-6; Knight 1985.
10. *History of the British Kings* and *The Life of Merlin* (Geoffrey of Monmouth) *Quest of The Holy Grail* (anonymous) plus a number of related or derivative sources.
11. My own recordings that apply these theories include records of the eighty-stringed psaltery (see Discography), music for Peter Redgrove's adaptation of *The Holy Sinner* (BBC Radio 3), music for BBC documentary film *Earth Magic* (1985), plus a number of works for classical guitar and small ensembles.
12. Godwin 1979.
13. Compare the very simple Tree of Life illustrated in our diagrams with those of Kircher (shown in Godwin) or of the nineteenth-century occult texts leading up to and including the publication of the *Golden Dawn* instructional material. For general illustrations, see Purce 1974.
14. Early accounts of the Otherworld frequently link the vision of a transcendent reality with musical symbolism and geometrical proportion. This runs through both sophisticated classical and later sources and material drawn from oral traditions. See Appendix 2 for the famous example set out by Plato.
15. Diamond 1979 gives a direct popular summary of some of the effects of music upon the organism.
16. See Diamond for a list of conductors' lifespans, (pages 95-6).
17. C. G. Jung made a number of studies of the mandala in the context of modern psychology. See Jung/Franz 1965 for a general definition in this respect.
18. See Kircher *Oedipus Aegyptiacus* for a complex diagram showing the relationship between the Seventy-Two Names of God. This includes a warning that such symbols are not to be used for superficial invocations. The tradition of such cautions is ancient and is not merely derived from orthodox religion, but from a desire on the part of authors, teachers, seers and metaphysicians to direct their students to the heart of the matter rather than the peripherals. (The Kircher illustration is shown in Godwin 1979.)
19. Translated J. J. Parry 1925.
20. Godwin 1986 provides a source book for references to Music, Magic and Mysticism, from the classical Greek period to the nineteenth century.

CHAPTER TWO

1. Godwin 1986; Chambers 1956; Stewart 1976.
2. See Gray 1969 for a lucid restatement of the Fourfold Cycle in magical symbolism. See Read 1961 for Alchemy; Mayo 1979 for astrological theory, also Mann 1979.
3. Out of the many composers who could be cited, the most outstanding include: Ralph Vaughan Williams; Percy Grainger; Igor Stravinsky; Bela Bartok; Charles Ives; Benjamin Britten. There is an important qualitative difference between the work of composers such as these and composers who 'arrange' folk melodies. The second category is far larger than the first.
4. Rudhyar 1982 gives an analysis of musical cultural growth, but omits to mention traditional music (folk or ethnic music) other than to state incorrectly that it is derived from plainsong (page 163). As has been proven very effectively by Fr Chambers (op. cit.), plainsong is derived from folksong. Otherwise Rudhyar is a perceptive and experienced modern author on music and consciousness.
5. The famous vocal works of John Dunstable, for example, are based upon astrological and Trinitarian calculations (died 1453).
6. See relevant entries in *Groves Dictionary* and the *Oxford Companion to Music*. An analysis is found in Rudhyar, pages 90-102. 'Temperament'.
7. Godwin 1986.
8. Stewart 1976; *Penguin Book of English Folksongs* 1959; Kennedy, 1984 (Ed.); Sharp 1960.
9. Chambers (op. cit.) Wagner; *History of Plainchant*.

CHAPTER THREE

1. This theory is epitomized in the works of Robert Fludd and Athanasius Kircher (see Godwin 1979). A summary of Renaissance theories is found in Walker: *Spiritual and Demonic Magic from Ficino to Campanella*. An Eastern parallel is stated in Govinda 1969.
2. 'Spirit. In Hebrew, Ruach; in Greek, Pneuma. In scripture the word Spirit is taken (1) For the Holy Ghost ... who inspired the Prophets, animates good men ... the Holy Ghost is called Spirit, being as it were breathed, and proceeding from the Father and Son who inspire and move our hearts by him ... ' *Cruden's Concordance*. 'Thereupon he straightway burst into tears, and drawing in the breath of Prophecy, spake, saying ... ' *Prophecies of Merlin*.
3. Chambers (op. cit.) quotes a number of direct statements from early Church Fathers and authorities which can hardly be denied or

refuted, dealing with application of peasant vocal calls to church use, singing and spiritual joy, and the relationship between singing and dancing. Chamber's evidence from early sources, more or less contemporary to the development of the Christian chant from social music, shows the remarkable prejudice displayed by 'classical' musicologists who repeatedly state that folk music is the result of peasants imitating plainchant. All music comes from folk music, from the music of the group consciousness attuned to the environment. (See Fig. 1.)

4. Purce 1974. Stewart 1985, chapter 8. Gray 1968.

5. Iamblichus, *Life of Pythagoras*, tr. Thomas Taylor 1818; Taylor, T. 1816/1972.

6. Berne, E. M. D., *Games People Play* (Penguin) is a good example of the Tree of Life polarity diagrams employed in popular psychology. It is interesting to see that this medical doctor does not know of the existence of the ancient psychology shown in Qabalah, or if he is aware of it, he chooses not to cite it as the original of his illustrations.

7. There are a large number of confused and mutually plagiarized books on the Tree of Life, mostly literary derivatives of Renaissance theosophy, or nineteenth-century studies such as those of the Order of the Golden Dawn. A brief examination of a few of these volumes will show how confused and contradictory the symbolism can be.

8. Chambers (op. cit.).

9. See Discography.

10. See relevant entries in *Groves/Oxford Companion to Music*.

11. See note 10 above.

12. Godwin 1979 reproduces a number of remarkable illustrations by Robert Fludd (1574-1637) which demonstrate this ancient harmonic theory.

13. See Discography.

14. 'What does singing a jubilation mean? It is the realization that words cannot express the inner music of the heart. For those who sing in the harvest field, or vineyard, or in work deeply occupying the attention, when they are overcome with joy at the words of the song, being filled with such exultation, the words fail to express their emotion, so leaving the syllables of the words, they drop into vowel sounds ... signifying that the heart is yearning to express what the tongue cannot utter.' St Augustine, commentary on Psalm 32.

15. See Discography for recordings that demonstrate this effect.

16. At the most opposite end of the spectrum, both in religion and in

music, we could cite the work of Olivier Messiaen, which (according to the composer himself in a telelvision interview broadcast in 1985) is derived partly from birdsong and structured through a system of tonal/elemental 'colours' that he employs for note-clusters or chords.

17. The confusing theory of the 'ancient Greek modes' found in many musical textbooks is derived from the (lost) scientific art of specific scales or modes inspiring specific qualities of consciousness. These were represented by the tribal characteristics of the Dorians, the Lydians, the Ionians and so forth. Language of this sort is symbolic and traditional, rather than literal and historic; endless musical confusion has arisen through taking the presumed symbolism of the 'Greek Modes' literally.

18. See Discography for examples. Also Govinda 1969 for the use of sacred sound in Tibetan monastic practice.

CHAPTER FOUR

1. See Rudhyar 1982, pages 72, 83, 100-1.
2. The simple experiment of putting an ear to the side of a harp, guitar or piano reveals a panoply of unsuspected sounds resonating within. This resonance is not present in electronic instruments, though an artificial enhancement is made by the use of reverberation, echo and digital storage and retrieval devices. A great deal of modern progressive electronic music merely states outwardly that which is heard in the heart of any acoustic resonating chamber, exteriorizing certain patterns, repetitions, rhythms and tonal sequences and playing them formally or recording them. This exteriorization is part of the cycle shown in Fig. 1, but also reveals the alienation between the consciousness of the modern musical mind and the very basic sounds of nature. Music is considered to be only the *expressed* and immediately audible structure; and with electronics this is indeed what it becomes.
3. Sharp 1960.
4. See *Augustine, De Musica*, quoted in Chambers, Chapter 3, pages 34-7.

CHAPTER FIVE

1. Read 1961; Atwood 1920; see also Appendix 3.
2. A number of notation or mnemonic systems persisted well into the eighteenth and nineteenth centuries which demonstrated the flexibility of systems other than the standard notation. There is still

controversy over the early systems of plainchant notation (see Chambers, Wagner) yet the parallels within oral tradition and early manuscripts are clear. 'Shape Notes' in which musical pitch is indicated by the digits of the hand or similar locations to aid memory are still found among dissenting sects; Irish harpers used a system involving the buttons of their coats; Scottish pipers had the *cantarach* system which was wiped out by English force of arms; in the *Scholar's Primer* (trans. C. Calder 1917) a number of fourteenth-century Irish texts relate a series of alphabets, some applied to the digits of the hand. A similar system is employed in China (Levis, J. Hazedel, *Chinese Musical Art*), and was directly used by the early Church, probably drawing upon pagan hand-location (Chironomic) systems of music. The failure to grasp this complex texture of musical symbolism is remarkable in standard musicology, as is the failure to grasp the remarkable power of the pre-literate musical memory.

3. Godwin 1986; Taylor, 1816, 1818.

4. See note 2 above.

5. See relevant entry in *Groves, The Oxford Companion to Music*, and note 18 to Chapter 3. See also Rudhyar 1982, pages 32, 84-8.

6. The image of Art as the Ape of Nature appears in a number of alchemical, Hermetic and metaphysical texts and illustrations, where it is suggestive of techniques (i.e. imitate nature, work holistically or organically and rhythmically) for harmony between the Worlds. The inverse of this image (the *demonic* inverse as the old philosophers would have termed it) is the theory that humankind is actually a type of ape shaped into its present form by an endless struggle with nature.

7. Godwin 1986.

8. See Fig. 5. The lyre has traditionally seven or eight strings, said to symbolize the Seven Planets. These open strings are tuned to a basic scale or mode, but the method of playing was derived by touching *harmonics* or *overtones*, a technique still used today on the harp and guitar, in which a light touch upon the surface of the plucked string elicits a series of clear notes (overtones) that are part of the fundamental note of the string. This very ancient method of playing remained active in Europe well into historical times with the *crwth* found in Wales, and the Scandinavian bowed harps. A small number of open strings can therefore produce a large range of true (i.e. untempered) harmonic intervals. Each string of the Lyre of Apollo will produce the 5th, 6th, 3rd and 7th *partials* as clear natural notes by lightly touching the surface in the appropriate place while plucking

with the other hand, or bowing. A further refinement of the technique enables the entire partial series to be sounded with varying degrees of clarity. In the lyre of eight strings, the eighth does not play the octave (as is commonly assumed) for this is found by the method described above. It is, instead, tuned *one semitone* below the octave; this tuning enables the player to render a fully chromatic series of partials, similar to the pattern of the modern keyboard, for the eighth string fills in the pitches that cannot be easily found on the main seven. (Examples of such tuning for experimental purposes would be: a/b/c/d/e/f/g/ a-flat; or c/d/e/f/g/a/b-flat/ b-natural, in which the 'odd' position becomes a natural rather than a flat note. This is a simplification of the ancient tuning, which also involved intervals smaller than a semi-tone, but serves to demonstrate the mysteries of the lyre for modern purposes. The lyre was invented by Hermes as a gift to Apollo.

9. Chambers (op. cit.).
10. Read 1961; Godwin 1979.
11. Knight 1978.
12. The modern restoration of so-called 'Druidism' need not be included in any serious study of Celtic lore, either in music or any other branch of traditional symbolism. It is significant that revival 'Druidism' (mainly a series of grotesque fabrications based upon pseudo-antiquarianism or pseudo-paganism) takes very little account of living current ethnic Celtic material.

CHAPTER SIX

1. Read 1961.
2. Gray 1969; Mann 1979; Mayo 1979. The standard astrological, alchemical and magical Elemental systems are different in several respects. The cyclical pattern of the magical circle is based upon a combination of Western traditions closely attuned to the Seasons and to the phases of human development. It is this system, with some specific variations, that is followed in our examples, as its spiralling property reflects the centrifugal nature of musical expansion from a primary tone. It should be stated fairly that the system has no 'known' origination and that it persists in various forms through many centuries. Specific authors merely represent individual collations, opinions, or fragments of research. The origin lies in human consciousness, and beyond that in the greater consciousness of Being. For an unusual modern example, see Dion Fortune, *The Cosmic Doctrine* (reprinted by Aquarian Press) which reflects a

combination of nineteenth-century theosophy with some highly original Hermetic concepts which the author drew from an intuitive inner source.

3. Theories regarding the nature of scales and their effect upon consciousness are not confined to esoteric studies or ancient traditions by any means. The nineteenth century saw the appearance of a refined *Tonic Sol Fa* system of music reading which had remarkable currency and popularity. Even today many popular song books are still published with the tonic solfa system beneath the regular score. In this system, which owes some of its theory to classical or Pythagorean antiquarianism, the Tonic is called the *firm or strong* note; the second the *rousing* note; the third the *calm or resolving* note; the fourth the *solemn or awe-inspiring* note; the fifth the *clarion of trumpet* note; the sixth the *sad or melancholic* note; and the seventh the *piercing* note. Many of these psychological terms are quite acceptably used by serious musicians or composers today.

4. Fludd; *Utriusque Cosmi . . . Historia* 1617 (History of the Macrocosm and the Microcosm). Illustrations include a 'Temple of Music' and a 'Cosmic Monochord'. These are reproduced in Godwin 1979.

5. *The Spiral of Octaves*: One revolution equals the interval of one *fourth* (notes 1-4 on a standard scale or CDEF). Two revolutions equal one *octave* (notes 1-8 or CDEFGABC). Eight revolutions (four octaves) returns the note C to the Element of Earth. This might be termed a *Great Cycle of Musical Elements*. A further three octaves would carry us to the limits of the human auditory range of seven octaves, assuming that our cycle begins on the lowest audible note. (In this example we are always using C as a theoretical lowest note or starting note merely for convenience; there is no implication of any particular C or fixed number of vibrations per second. For the actual acoustics of the human auditory range see various reference works listed in the Bibliography.) Our extension or centrifugal expansion of seven octaves brings us once more to the note C, or number 57 from a note C as the first number. The C notes (1, 8, 15, 22, 29, 36, 43, 50, 57) rise in a sunwise or clockwise rotation: C1 Earth; C8 Air; C15 Fire; C22 Water; C29 Earth and onwards to C57. The spiral of ascending notes in the mode or scale, however, runs starwise or anti-clockwise, shown in our diagram of the Spiral of Octaves. Because our example is deliberately limited to the basic modern major scale and its adjustment or temperament, no indication is shown of (a) the sequence of fifths adjusted by the necessary sharps, or (b) the actual acoustic nature of the expanding fifths which actually exceeds

the number of corresponding octaves. (See Rudhyar Chapter 7 for a discussion of this relationship between fifths and octaves.)

CHAPTER SEVEN

1. A modern restatement of this concept, with quite different emphasis and background, may be found in the Alexander technique, where conscious control of the body is practised with far-reaching effect. See Barlow 1973.
2. Jaynes 1976; Onians 1973. See also a short summary of the origins of the word *thymos* in Diamond 1979, appendix II, page 128.
3. Stewart, 1986.
4. It is worth noting that the general concept of psychic power, power or tonal centres, predates modern scientific definition of bio-electrical energy by many centuries.
5. This derives from Talmudic or biblical tradition in which *Adam* means one made of red earth or dust. Much confusion has been generated in esoteric publications through the Church equating Earth/Nature with evil or corruption, a concept quite alien to the Mysteries or the genuine traditions of spiritual development worldwide.
6. See Jung 1968, 1953, 1959, for modern psychological theories on the imagination. It must be stressed that the use of creative imagination in meditation, magic and similar artistic sciences is not identical to the psychological interpretation and use.
7. Steiner 1910.
8. Stewart 1985, page 47, 130; 1986 chapter 2; Steiner op. cit.
9. Rudhyhar 1982 on the properties of scales; Govinda 1969 on the reiteration of the mantram AUM through the worlds.

CHAPTER EIGHT

1. The most famous 'word of power' is JHVH deriving from orthodox Hebrew tradition and from unorthodox Hebrew mysticism. This Name, however, has roots in the psychic-spiritual foundation of magic, and a number of other non-Hebraic god names share similar sounds and traditional properties. Alchemical and Hermetic illustrations abound with examples of the Name, both in musical and non-musical contexts. For examples see Read 1961.
2. A less published Name, also derived from Hebraic tradition in the general literature of the occult revival, is AHIH; a breathing sound. Once again it must be stressed that such words are primal sounds

or tones of consciousness, there is no religious or racial or hierarchical authority attached to them; the power is inherent in the word and its harmonic link to intuitions about reality, not in the literary or religious or superstitious sources and usages. We should also be aware that such 'words' are not only indicative of higher and altered states of consciousness, *but are direct expressions of such states.* The curious phenomenon of 'speaking with tongues' is known worldwide, and even has a Christian authoritarian tradition derived from the New Testament. This spontaneous mode of utterance, which is often musically pitched, is an individual or group psychic manifestation (as sound) which reflects the greater utterance of the Creative Word. In most cases speaking with tongues is a purely transitory phenomenon, relating only to the immediate cult or group use and with no communicable 'words' for any further use. Words of Power, however, have an enduring and undying cycle of meaning; they encapsulate and express a higher consciousness and a fundamental consciousness simultaneously.

3. The orthodox biblical reference to Spirit moving upon the face of the deep are merely one set of examples of an enduring body of symbolism. We could cite other Western sources which are non-Christian, such as the Finnish Kalevala, *a virgin daughter of Air (Ilmatar) descends to float upon the great waters until (after 700 years) a bird sent by a male deity (Ukko) lays seven eggs upon her knees. Out of these eggs the world (or Worlds) hatch.*

4. See Govinda 1969, page 23. In Tibetan Buddhism the syllable OM is defined as three units: A-U-M. Each unit or letter equates with a plane of consciousness: 'A' waking consciousness; 'U' dream consciousness; 'M' consciousness during deep sleep. The unified syllable AUM (OM) represents cosmic consciousness. In Eastern monastic practice, as in Western, sacred words are uttered *musically*, upon drawn out and regulated tones. A word of power or seed-syllable means very little if it is merely spoken conversationally, and even less if it is merely read about without actual involvement or experience on the part of the reader. The obvious similarities between the Buddhist, Hebrew and Western magical traditions are emphatically *not* a matter of literary or historical derivation; their essential unity demonstrates a property of human consciousness as it relates to the mysteries of the unknown origin of Being.

5. Stewart 1985, pages 105-9.

6. Govinda, op. cit., page 253 for a map of AUM progressing through the metaphysical worlds and acting upon their inhabitants. This

type of symbolism is well known in the West, in orthodox forms such the power ascribed to the name of Jesus (to which all beings in all worlds show respect due to his divine nature and more specifically due to the 'Harrowing of Hell') or in magical traditions where certain utterances, pitches, tones or shapes (Names) will contact beings in other dimensions or the inner worlds. We can find a rather simplistic but viable parallel in modern psychology, in which the musical keys unlock areas of the individual consciousness and reveal the contents, often manifesting as imaginary beings or persons intimately attuned to those same areas. The passage of a word such as OM or JESUS, however, is of a different order and value to that of minor psychic restructuring. The first are of enduring cosmic significance, while the second are merely personal and ephemeral. If the greater 'names' 'words' or 'seed syllables' are applied musically to the individual psyche, we are working towards an opening and a union between general and transcendent consciousness.

7. Cruden: 'Signifies in Hebrew true, faithful, certain. It is made use of likewise to affirm any thing and was an affirmation used often by our Saviour' (Concordance 1817). AMEN has specific and repeated use on both Old and New Testaments in a manner that shows it was employed as a word of truth or word of power. (John 3.3, 5/2Cor.1.20/Rev. 3.14/Isa.65.16/Rev. 5.14, etc.)

APPENDIX ONE

1. It has been constant practice throughout this book not to cite specific pieces of music, particularly in negative terms. Unhealthy or depressing serious music usually includes works which reflect intellectual or 'arty' contrivance for the sake of fame, grants or ephemeral fashion at the most superficial level, or deep obsessions and mental imbalance at the most significant. Many such works have an unhealthy attraction which is lessened and balanced by use of the simple rules shown in the Appendix.

The novelty period for 'avant-garde' and 'new wave' or 'new age' music has not passed (1987), and we should be especially wary of self-acclaimed progressive or spiritual music. Most of this material is a refined variant of pop product (see Chapter 1) and may be distinguished by the development of musically alert consciousness. The use of Elemental tones and calls to awaken the psyche should enable the reader to refresh his or her musical taste and intuition;

it would be quite irrelevant in a book of this sort to print lists of apparently 'good' or 'bad' recordings or musical works. This method merely returns us to the tossing ocean of general musical use; what is required is to transmute this vast chaotic sea down into a transformative essence — the musically purified elements of the psyche.

APPENDIX FIVE

1. If we delved deeper into the science of acoustics, we could make some fine distinctions between our reiterated notes throughout the Tree of Life: the solution of tempering a scale enables us to use the notes in a symbolic manner that avoids this important but complex set of distinctions; in an untempered scale our various notes will be of differing rates of vibration (although called by the same letter of the alphabet) *depending upon the direction by which we approach them.* This important micro-tonal difference is the key to a very ancient method of chanting and playing music, and is still found in the sacred and magical music of the East today as a tradition in which the metaphysical elements or systems are only partly understood. In our example, the Proportional Tree of Life, a guide is shown which may be fully defined by an acoustic table or set of calculations, giving a guide to performance and intonation of metaphysical microtonal music. (See relevant entries in *Groves* or *Oxford Companion* for subjects such as temperament, chromatic scales, micro-tones, quarter tones, intervals, etc.)

2. This extract is concerned with operations of ritual magic and their effect upon consciousness. It does not, as such, give a musical system for the individual to use in meditation or progressive development, but deals directly with certain magical and metaphysical topics and methods. The author is restating a very hallowed ancient tradition where people gather together and use music in group work to change their consciousness and to change the outer world by a musical vehicle that draws energies from an inner world. In pagan traditions this type of method was widespread in the Mysteries, while in Christian use it incorporates early communal singing, plainchant, and of course the modern use of hymn singing. Musical applications to consciousness are still being developed today, and the system quoted is only one of a series of modern researches into music and changing consciousness. These researches are made by separate groups or individuals, but are all based upon Elemental rotations of music and energy; most important is not the content but the

fact that the material is *practical* and not merely receptive or theoretical. Modern experimenters with altered consciousness are developing new ways of using music. The days of listening to selected recordings or reiterating religious chant are over.

Bibliography

Attwood, A. (1920) *A Suggestive Enquiry into the Hermetic Mystery*, Belfast.

Barlow, W. (1973) *The Alexander Principle*, London.

Berne, E. M. D. (1970) *Games People Play*, Harmondsworth.

Boethius, *De Musica*.

Bowra, C. M. (1962) *Primitive Song*, London.

Chamberlain, D. S. 'Philosophy of Music in the *Consolatio* of Boethius' (*Speculum* (1970) pages 80-97).

Chambers, Fr. G. B. (1956) *Folksong-Plainsong*, London.

Diamond, J. (1979) *Behavioral Kinesiology*, New York.

Erickson, R. (1975) *Sound Structure in Music*, Berkeley.

Fortune, D. (1966) *The Mystical Qabalah*, London.

Fortune, D. (1976) *The Cosmic Doctrine*, Wellingborough.

Gantz, J. (trans.) (1976) *The Mabinogion*, Harmondsworth.

Godwin, J. (1979) *Robert Fludd*, London.

Godwin, J. (1979) *Athanasius Kircher*, London.

Godwin, J. (1986) *Music, Magic Mysticism*, London.

Govinda, Lama A. (1969) *Foundations of Tibetan Mysticism*, London.

Gray, W. G. (1968) *The Ladder of Lights*, Teddington.

Gray, W. G. (1969) *Magical Ritual Methods*, Teddington.

Hamel, P. M. (1976) *Through Music to the Self*, Salisbury.

Hopkins, A. J. (1934) *Alchemy, Child of Greek Philosophy*, New York.

Jaynes, J. (1976) *The Origins of Consciousness in the Bicameral Mind*, Boston.

Jung, C. G. (1953) *Two Essays on Analytical Psychology*, London.

Jung, C. G. (1968) *Civilisation in Transition*, London.

Jung, C. G.(1959) *Psychological Types*, London.

Jung, C. G. (1953) *Psychology and Alchemy*, London.

Jung, C. G./Franz (1965) *Man and His Symbols*, London.

Jung, C. G. and Wilhelm, R. (1965) *The Secret of the Golden Flower*, London.

Kathi, M. (1970) *Music of the Spheres and the Dance of Death*, Princeton.

Kennedy, P. (1984) *Folksongs of Britain and Ireland*, London, New York.

Knight, G. (1978) *A History of White Magic*, London.

Knight, G. (1983) *The Secret Tradition in Arthurian Legend*, Wellingborough.

Lilly, W. (ed. Zadkiel) (1913) *An Introduction to Astrology*, London.

MacCana, P. (1975) *Celtic Mythology*, London.

Mann, A. T. (1979) *The Round Art*, London.

Matarasso, P. (trans.) (1969) *The Quest of the Holy Grail*, Harmondsworth.

Matthews, J. and C. (1985-6) *The Western Way*, Vols. 1 and 2, London.

Mayo, J. (1979) *Astrology*, London.

Onians, R. B. (1973) *The Origins of European Thought*, New York.

Parry, J. J. (1925) (trans.) *Vita Merlini*, Illinois.

Portnoy, J. (1954) *The Philosopher and Music*, New York.

Portnoy, J. (1963) *Music in the Life of Man*, New York.

Priestley, M. (1975) *Music Therapy in Action*, London.

Purce, J. (1974) *The Mystic Spiral*, London.

Read, J. (1939/1961) *Prelude to Chemistry*, London.

Rees, A. and B. (1961) *Celtic Heritage*, London.

Regardie, I. (1968) *The Tree of Life*, New York.

Regardie, I. (1937-40/1984) *The Golden Dawn*, Chicago/New York.

Ross, A. (1974) *Pagan Celtic Britain*, London.

Rudhyar, D. (1982) *The Magic of Tone and the Art of Music*, Boulder, Col.

Schneider, M. (1957) in Wellesz *Ancient and Oriental Music*, Oxford.

Scott, C. (1958) *Music*, London.

Sharp, C. (1960) *English Folksongs from the Southern Appalachians*, London.

Spitzer, L. (1963) *Classical and Christian Ideas of World Harmony*, Baltimore.

Steiner, R. (1907) *The Occult Significance of the Blood*, London.

Steiner, R. (1910) *Initiation and its Results*, London.

Stewart, R. J. (1986) *The Prophetic Vision of Merlin*, London.

Stewart, R. J. (1976) *Where is Saint George?* Bradford-on-Avon.

Stewart, R. J. (1985) *The UnderWorld Initiation*, Wellingborough.

Tart, C. T. (1975) *Transpersonal Psychologies*, New York/London.

Taylor, Th. (1816/1972) *The Theoretic Arthimetic of the Pythagoreans*, London/New York.

Taylor, Th. (trans.) *The Republic* (of Plato) London.

Thorpe, L. (trans.) (1966) *The History of the Kings of Britain*, Harmondsworth.

Vaughan Williams, R. and Lloyd, A. L. (eds.) *Penguin Book of English Folksongs* (1959) Harmondsworth.

Vogel, M. (1954) *Die Zahl Sieben in der spekulativen Musiktheorie*, Bonn.

West, J. A. and Toonder, G. (1970) *The Case of Astrology*, London.

A Short Discography

There are thousands of recordings of ethnic, religious and composed music that derive from conscious or unconscious methods of altering awareness through musical patterns or tone qualities.

As we are primarily concerned with simple musical calls and tones for practical work, the following recordings are merely a short sample of music on disc or tape that incorporate traditions or inspirational qualities of altered consciousness and enlivened imagination. This list is not definitive, authoritative or in any way superior to any other list; it does not comprise a work-programme, though free visualization to selected recordings can be extremely rewarding.

Atrium Musical de Madrid, *Music of Ancient Greece*, HM 1015.

BBC Records, *Chinese Classical Music*, REGK 1M.

Baron, Jean, and Anneix, Christian, *Bombarde et Biniou Koz* (traditional Breton music), Arfolk SB 357.

Claddagh, *The Drones and the Chanters* (traditional Irish piping), CC11.

Dunstable, J., *Motets*, Hilliard Ensemble, HMV 1467 031.

Gerwig, Walter, *Lute Music*, J. S. Bach, Oryx BACH 1202.

Gregorian Chant, *Ave Maria*, Philips Festivo 6570 154.

Hildegard of Bingen, Abbess, *A Feather on the Breath of God*, Gothic Voices, Hyperion A66039.

Lassus, O., *Lagrimi di San Pietro*, Consort of Musicke, Oiseau-Lyre DSLO 574.

Scriabin, A., *Symphonies 1-3*, Melodiya 80030 XHK.

Stewart, R. J., *Music and the Elemental Psyche* (recordings by R. J. Stewart are available from Sulis Music, BCM Box 3721, London WC1 3XX).

Stewart, R. J., *The Fortunate Isle* (a suite for psaltery and ensemble).

Stewart, R. J., *The Journey to the Underworld/Psaltery Music*.

Stewart, R. J., *The Unique Sound of the Psaltery.*
Stravinsky, I., *Le Sacre du Printemps* (conducts his work) CBS 72054.
Tantric Rituals, *Music of Tibet*, Library of Congress Recordings.
Watkins, David, *Music for Harp*, RCA 5087.
Vaughan Williams, R., *A Pastoral Symphony*, RCA SB6861 (LSC 3281).
Vaughan Williams, R., *The Sons of Light*, Lyrita SRCS 125.

The following record labels carry extensive lists of ethnic and unusual music:

Ar Hooli, Folkways, Harmonia Mundi, Le Chant du Monde, Lyrachord, Ocara, Rounder and Topic.

Many source recordings of traditional music worldwide are found in the USA Library of Congress, the BBC sound archives and university departments specializing in music, anthropology, folklore and comparative religion.

Index

159

160